30-Day Ketogenic Meal Plan:

The Ultimate Keto Meal Plan to Lose Weight and Be Healthy in 30 Days

Tyler MacDonald

Table of Contents

Introduction

First off, thank you for choosing 30-Day Ketogenic Meal Plan 2021. This is your first step along the path of weight loss and a healthy lifestyle. I'm sure this isn't an easy first step either. The worthwhile steps never are, but you took it.

It's tough when you have a busy schedule and life to find time to make smart choices. When you add in a new diet, that makes life even more difficult. The thing is, it doesn't have to be that way. With some careful planning, you can lose weight, get healthy, and still accomplish everything else that you want.

The first thing you have to do is figure out what you can and cannot eat when following a ketogenic diet. Then, you find a bunch of recipes, calculate your macros, and create a meal plan. That's it. Once you have come up with that meal plan, you write down a grocery list of things you need and get it.

But, I understand it's easier said than done. It can be frustrating to do all of that on your own, especially if you follow a new diet. That's what this book is here to help you. You will find all of the recipes you need and tips on creating your own meal plan. The best part, though, is there is a 30-day plan within these pages.

In those 30 days, you will lose weight, reach ketosis, and see amazing results. You will also get a good understanding of what it's like to be on a ketogenic diet. That means when those 30 days are up, you will feel confident enough to create your own meal plans so that you stick with the diet and continue to get healthy.

The meal plan is going to jumpstart your journey. Plus, you will find more recipes that you can use for the meal plans you will create. That means this book contains more than just the recipes used in the 30-day meal plan.

I am very excited for you to continue on your weight loss journey. You will discover a lot about yourself along the way, and I'm certain you will enjoy every minute of it. I want you to commit to yourself right now that you will follow this 30-day meal plan. Trust me; you won't regret it.

The Basics

The ketogenic diet isn't just a popular diet of today. It is easy to stick with and help you feel better overall. With this diet, you eat low carbs, moderate protein, and high fats. By doing this, your body learns to burn your fat stores instead of carbs for fuel. Burning fat creates more energy to get you through your day. You will soon have more energy than you have ever had in your life. This diet helps you lose weight and get rid of fat.

Your body's fat stores get converted into fatty acids that are used in the liver. They then get pushed through the body as ketones that are used as glucose sugar rather than artificial sugar.

This allows the body to grow and repair itself better. It also gives the body more calories to burn for energy without having to eat as much.

The most important thing you need to know about this diet is the way ketosis works. Ketosis is the main structure of this diet.

Once the body gets into the state of ketosis, it means the body will break down the fat stores to give your body the energy it needs. This means the body is giving itself a way to use the fats you eat rather than depending on the carbs you eat. You might still be wondering what the ketogenic diet is. Let's dig a bit deeper and find out.

This diet was developed in the 1920s to treat epilepsy. This diet stopped being used when pharmaceutical companies developed anti-seizure medication. Now, 70 years later, doctors have rediscovered it as a better alternative than medicine. It has become more popular and is constantly receiving attention in the media for the numerous problems it can treat.

The Principles

When you learn more about keto-friendly foods and are used to living a keto life, it will be easy for you to know how much and what you need to eat. Here is what your daily macros, fats, proteins, and carbs need to look like.

- *Carbohydrates*

Everybody's carbs tolerance will be different. The challenge is finding your "ideal" intake. When starting this diet, begin with a very low level of carbs to make sure you get into ketosis fast. This is the state where your body makes the ketones. A goal would be around 20 grams of carbs each day. The best way to measure blood ketones is with a blood ketone meter. These let you measure your ketones after three days of following the keto lifestyle. You can also use urine strips to measure your ketones, but these aren't as accurate. Begin adding carbs around five grams per week until you can barely detect extremely low levels of ketones. This is the most reliable way to figure out your limit of carbs. You can easily find urine strips or blood ketone meters online.

- *Protein*

How much protein you should consume can be figured out by activity level and body weight. More active people will need more protein during the day than those who have a sedentary lifestyle. A better estimate for people who have high body fat could be figured by subtracting the amount of protein you eat from the lean body mass. This is figured by subtracting body fat from body weight.

Eating enough protein is great for building or preserve muscle mass. If you eat too much protein, you could knock yourself out of ketosis since your body converts excess protein into glycogen.

- *How Much Protein?*

If you know your weight in pounds, just multiply that by 0.6 to get the lowest grams of protein you need to consume every day. To find the largest amount, you have to figure out your weight in grams and multiply that by your weight in pounds. If you know your weight in kilograms, multiply that by 1.3 or 2.2. This rule will apply to most people, but athletes will have higher protein requirements. You need to eat the least amount of protein to keep from losing muscle mass while dieting. If you are very active, you need to eat as close to your top limit as possible.

- *Fat: 60 to 75 percent*

Your fat intake makes up the rest of your energy needs. It is the filler to your energy requirements. Fat intake will be different for everyone, and it depends on what your goals are. You don't even need to count your calories or fat intake while following a keto diet because, normally, you won't overeat. When you eat foods that are low carb, a moderate amount of protein, and high in fats will keep you feeling fuller longer. Studies show that fats and protein are the most filling nutrients, while carbs aren't. Fat gives you a lot of energy without spiking your insulin. This is why you shouldn't have any cravings while following this diet. You shouldn't suffer and mood or energy swings like you would on a low fat, calorie restricted diet.

Guidelines

Here are some great ways to help you stay in ketosis and get the most from your ketogenic diet. These tips will help you through the "keto flu." In the first few days or weeks while your body transitions into ketosis, you might feel dizzy, sluggish, or tired.

- *Macros*

You need to be sure you stick with your macros. The normal 10 percent carbs, 20 percent protein, and 70 percent fats should be followed simply because it works. If you eat too many carbs, you aren't going to be burning fat. If you eat too much protein, it isn't going to get burned because you aren't using it. If you don't eat enough fats, you aren't going to feel full. All of this will add up to less energy. These ratios let you eat whole foods to get into ketosis, and this includes lots of leafy green vegetables that help break down meats.

- *Electrolytes*

Make sure you keep plenty of electrolytes in your system. Electrolytes are minerals in the blood that keep the body hydrated and help the muscles and nerves work in unison. When your body begins producing ketones, it will flush out more water, which depletes the body's supply of electrolytes. This means you need to increase the amount of salt in your diet since your body can't retain sodium. Many keto followers fix this problem by drinking bouillon or bone broth each day. This is especially true during the first few weeks on this diet while the body gets adjusted. If you begin to feel achy while your body goes through carb withdrawals, bouillon will help. Other keto followers will take magnesium supplements, too.

- *Water*

You need to drink more water than normal. Everybody says you need to drink water, but no one takes it seriously until they get kidney stones. Drinking no less than 64 ounces of water every day is going to make your body feel hydrated, full, and clean. It also helps keep your bowels working correctly. If you are looking to lose weight while on this diet, water will help you with this, too.

- *Track Your Eating*

You need to measure what you eat. By doing this, it can turn this diet into a game. You can find apps that will help you measure your macros and track your meals daily. A specific app called Quip helps you make shopping lists. It has checkmarks that let you use your shopping list over and over again.

- *Calories*

You need to make sure you eat all your calories. You can't do a low-calorie diet along with a ketogenic diet. If you do this, your body won't be able to fuel itself. Fat is now what fuels your body. Without eating the correct amounts, you are going to feel hungry, and you aren't going to lose any weight. Most people who follow the keto diet eat between 1,800 and 2,000 calories each day. You might realize that eating less isn't going to help you lose weight; it might actually stall any weight loss. You can't binge eat, either. You aren't going to lose weight if you eat 5,000 calories each day.

- *Healthy Fats*

You need to have a lot of healthy fats on hand. Fat is considered a bad word in society today. What most people don't realize is there are a lot of good fats out there. Cook your foods in coconut oil or olive oil. Stay away from oils such as corn, soybean, sunflower seed, and vegetable oils. These are all high in omega 6s that cause inflammation. They can actually destroy the omega 3s that are in your body.

- *Whole Foods*

You need to buy whole foods and stay away from anything that says "low carb" on the label. If you look at the label on anything labeled as "low carb", you are going to be shocked at what is in them. Most of it is additives that can't be pronounced. You get to control what goes into your body when you make your meals at home and stick to eating whole foods.

Creating a Meal Plan

If you would like to know how to make your own meal plan, here is a guide you can follow:

1. Make a draft

Think about what foods you enjoy eating and see if they are on the approved list. Go from there and create your own diet plan. Remember to include lots of healthy fats, a moderate amount of protein, and low carbs.

2. Check

Go through the recipes you've put into your meal plan to see if the carbs, proteins, and fats match your body weight. If they don't, readjust the meal plan.

3. Research

Before you begin making a meal plan, research various keto meal plans and see how they measure up. Make sure you go through this whole guide since you don't want to jump in blind.

4. Revise

Make any changes you need to make and revise any recipes that need to be made better.

5. Discuss

If you are not sure about anything, talk with an expert. If you still aren't sure, follow the meal plan below or ask other people who have done this diet.

6. Repair

Look for any improvements that are needed and make any changes that you need to. Be sure it matches your percentage needs of 10/20/70.

7. Follow through

If you are ready, let's get started.

Here are some tips that will help you be successful when following your meal plan:

- Realize that diets aren't good for everyone. Be sure your diet plan and recipes match your requirements. Make any adjustments and make the portions smaller if needed. If you go over your protein intake, don't worry too much. Just adjust and keep moving forward. If you realize your diet doesn't include enough fats, this can be easily remedied by adding oil or butter to meals.

- Substitute lamb, pork, and fish for each other in recipes because their nutritional values are similar.

- Don't eat unless you are hungry. If you don't feel hungry at mealtime, don't eat. It is perfectly fine to skip a meal.

- Try skipping snacks. You should feel full from your three main meals. If you don't, keep some keto-friendly snacks at hand.

- Swap meals: You can swap up your meals during the day. You can eat breakfast for dinner or lunch for breakfast or dinner for lunch. What you eat depends on you.

- Cook your meal. When you cook your own meals, you can control what goes into them. Freeze any uneaten portions or save half and eat it later.

While you adapt to the ketogenic lifestyle and make your own meal plans, watch out for the following. These are usually sold with fillers and added sugars. Check labels before you buy products, and don't forget to calculate your net carbs by subtracting fiber from the total carbs. You want to purchase items that have low net carbs.

- Sliced cheese, especially American, can have around three carbs for each slice. Stick with shredded cheese that contains no fillers. You will be eating less than one carb per serving.

- Salad dressing: these might have a lot of sugar in them. Look for ones that have around one net carb for each serving.

- Sugar-free: Just because something is labeled as "sugar-free" doesn't mean it will be low carb. Anything that is labeled as "gluten-free" will never equal low carb. Low carb doesn't mean it will be ketogenic. You could find 20 to 30 carbs in a bagel that is labeled as low carb.

- Frozen burgers: Most frozen foods use fillers and could carry between three and five carbs per burger. If you made them yourself, it could be zero carbs.

- Deli foods: Grocery stores make it easy to walk in and grab a quick bite to eat. Even though these are made each day, they usually include breading and sugars you won't be able to see just by looking at them.

- Whey protein: This powder might be very high in sugar. Check the label to find some no or low-carb varieties.

- Coconut milk: This contains good fats but does contain about one net carb for unsweetened. The sweetened variety has about nine carbs per serving.

- Tomato sauce: When looking for tomato sauce in the grocery store, you will see there will be anywhere between 10 and 20 net carbs in each serving. Try to find ones that don't have any added sugars and are less than four net carbs for each serving.

- Dairy products: Again, look at the labels. Most cream cheese, sour cream, and heavy whipping cream will have around two to three net carbs for each serving. Organic brands won't have any carbs or under one net carb.

- Peanut butter: Most brands of peanut butter will contain a lot of sugar. Find a brand that has low net carbs. The organic brands will contain very low or no sugar.

Sticking with the Diet

There are various ways to help you stick with a diet. Most people will give up after some time, and it is mainly because normal diets make them give up foods that they like eating. The keto diet requires you to give up many foods you like, but this is mainly carbs. This makes it easier to stay on and maintain. Here are some tips to make sure you stay healthy while following this diet for a long time.

- Don't let yourself get hungry. Many times, if you let yourself get too hungry, you will eat carb-heavy foods that fill you up fast. It can make you have poor judgment when it comes to deciding what you want to eat. You might pick something that won't be good for your new lifestyle.

- Eat vegetables or berries for a snack. If you get hungry between meals, have a handful of nuts, berries, or veggies for a snack. These are nutritious and healthy options that take the place of cupcakes or cookies.

- Make sure you get enough sleep. Studies show that you eat more when you are tired. This produces a hormone that will trick you into thinking you are hungry.

- Drink water. Water doesn't just flush toxins out of your body, but it keeps you hydrated, too. It could also distract you from whatever craving you might be having.

- Find recipes you want to try that are in your diet's guidelines. When you have various foods to taste and sample, it will be easier to stick with your diet since you are eating a variety of foods, and it won't become boring.

- Try new things and create new recipes. Use foods you know you can eat and try to make new recipes. Being able to play around and experiment will keep your food interesting.

- Create an achievable goal. Having clear goals will motivate you to make sure you reach them.

- Take vitamins and supplements if you need them. Talk with your doctor first if you think you have a deficiency. Then if they say it is fine, take a supplement

- Find an accountability partner. If you have somebody you have to report to and will support your progress, it will help you stay on track. Find somebody who will support you mentally as well as physically.

30-Day Meal Plan

The 30-Day Meal Plan is broken down into four weeks. Every day has a snack option. Now, you can choose to eat the snack between lunch and dinner, or you can have the snack as a dessert after dinner. If there is a day where you don't feel like you want a snack or dessert, that's perfectly fine. You don't have to eat one.

Week One	Breakfast	Lunch	Snack	Dinner
Day 1	Avocado Milkshake	Chicken Wraps	Cinnamon Smoothie	Cauliflower Mac & Cheese
Day 2	Granola	Cauliflower Soup	Blueberry Smoothie	Turkey Meatloaf
Day 3	Peanut Butter Smoothie	Grilled Salmon with Asparagus	Dark Chocolate	Lettuce Wrap Cheeseburger
Day 4	Cream Cheese Pancakes	Cauliflower Soup (leftovers)	Vanilla Ice Cream	Grilled Salmon with Asparagus (leftovers)
Day 5	Keto Coffee	Turkey Meatloaf (leftovers)	Bacon Deviled Eggs	Haddock
Day 6	Lemon Smoothie	Haddock (leftovers)	Dark Chocolate	Pork Loin with Mustard Sauce
Day 7	Bacon and Eggs	Taco Salad	Parmesan Chips	Pork Loin with Mustard Sauce (leftovers)

Week Two	Breakfast	Lunch	Snack	Dinner
Day 8	Breakfast Bake	Crab Salad Avocado	Kale Chips	Zucchini Gratin
Day 9	Peanut Butter Smoothie	Tuna Salad	Parmesan Chips	Thai Chicken Soup
Day 10	Keto Coffee	Zucchini Gratin (leftovers)	Mixed Berries	Bacon Cheese Burger Soup
Day 11	Breakfast Bake (leftovers)	Thai Chicken Soup (leftovers)	Dark Chocolate	Tuna Salad (leftovers)
Day 12	Green Smoothie	Chicken Bacon Burger	Parmesan Chips	Lamb with Sun-Dried Tomatoes
Day 13	Keto Coffee	BLT Salad	Brownies	Thai Lettuce Wrap
Day 14	Avocado and Eggs	Lamb with Sun-Dried Tomatoes (leftovers)	Brownies	Bacon Cheese Burger Soup (leftovers)

Week Three	Breakfast	Lunch	Snack	Dinner
Day 15	Berry Shake	Salmon Salad	Nut Butter and Veggies	Cheesy Broccoli Soup
Day 16	Breakfast Crème	Feta Salad	Cinnamon Smoothie	Cauliflower Soup
Day 17	Lemon Smoothie	Cheesy Broccoli Soup (leftovers)	Brownies	Salmon Salad (leftovers)
Day 18	Avocado and Eggs	Bolognese Zoodles	Dark Chocolate	Cauliflower Soup (leftovers)
Day 19	Cream Cheese Pancakes	Grilled Salmon with Asparagus	Pork Rinds	Cheeseburger
Day 20	Keto Coffee	Cheesy Broccoli Soup (leftovers)	Bacon Fat Bombs	Chicken Bacon Burger
Day 21	Keto Coffee	Feta Salad (leftovers)	Parmesan Chips	Grilled Salmon with Asparagus (leftovers)

Week Four	Breakfast	Lunch	Snack	Dinner
Day 22	Green Smoothie	Zesty Tilapia	Blueberry Muffin	Tri-Tip
Day 23	Peanut Butter Smoothie	Avocado Pesto Zoodles	Pecan Peanut Butter Bars	Sausage Casserole
Day 24	Keto Coffee	Roasted Chicken Thighs with Veggies	Beef Jerky	Zesty Tilapia (leftovers)
Day 25	Chia Berry Smoothie Bowl	Avocado Pesto Zoodles (leftovers)	Peanut Butter Smoothie	Sausage Crust Pizza
Day 26	Blueberry Muffin (leftover)	Sausage Casserole (leftovers)	Peanut Butter Cookies	Garlic Parmesan Salmon
Day 27	Keto Coffee	Zesty Tilapia (leftovers)	Dark Chocolate	Coconut Lime Skirt Steak
Day 28	Bacon and Eggs	Turkey Avocado Salad	Blueberry Muffin	Roasted Chicken Thighs with Veggies (leftovers)
Day 29	Keto Coffee	Garlic Parmesan Salmon (leftovers)	Peanut Butter Smoothie	Coconut Lime Skirt Steak (leftovers)
Day 30	Goat Cheese Omelet	Turkey Avocado Salad (leftovers)	Peanut Butter Cookies	Creamy Butter Chicken

Breakfast

Avocado Milkshake

This recipe makes 1 serving and contains 437 calories; 43 grams fat; 4 grams protein; 10 grams net carbohydrates per serving

What You Need

- Ice cubes, 5

- Liquid stevia, 5 drops

- Unsweetened coconut milk, .5 c

- Avocado, .5

What to Do

1. Simply place the ingredients in your blender and mix until it reaches a smooth consistency.

Granola

This recipe makes 8 servings and contains 391 calories; 38 grams fat; 10 grams protein; 4 grams net carbohydrates per serving

What You Need

- Sunflower seeds, 1 c

- Sliced almonds, 1 c

- Nutmeg, .5 tsp.

- Cinnamon, 1 tsp.

- Liquid stevia, 10 drops

- Shredded unsweetened coconut, 2 c

- Melted coconut oil, .5 c

- Walnuts, .5 c

- Pumpkin seeds, .5 c

What to Do

1. Start by placing your oven on 250. Place parchment paper on two baking sheets and place to the side.

2. Toss the walnuts, pumpkin seeds, sunflower seeds, almonds, and shredded coconut together.

3. Blend together the nutmeg, cinnamon, stevia, and coconut oil.

4. Pour the coconut oil over the nut mixture and toss everything together using your hands. Make sure everything is well coated.

5. Spread the granola out between the two baking sheets.

6. Slide this in the oven and let it bake for an hour. Every 10-15 minutes, the mixture needs to be stirred to make sure that it browns evenly on all sides.

7. Pour the granola in a bowl and allow it to cool off before storing.

Peanut Butter Smoothie

This recipe makes 2 servings and contains 486 calories; 40 grams fat; 30 grams protein; 6 grams net carbohydrates per serving

What You Need

- Ice cubes, 3

- Peanut butter, 2 tbsp.

- Chocolate protein powder, 1 scoop

- Coconut cream, .75 c

- Water, 1 c

What to Do

1. Simply place the ingredients in a blender and mix until it reaches a smooth consistency. Divide into two glasses and serve.

Cream Cheese Pancakes

This recipe makes 1 serving and contains 365 calories; 29 grams fat; 17 grams protein; 5 grams net carbohydrates per serving

What You Need

- Packet stevia

- Cinnamon, .5 tsp.

- Coconut flour, 1 tbsp.

- Cream cheese, 2 oz.

- Eggs, 2

What to Do

1. Place everything in a bowl and beat everything together until it forms a smooth batter.

2. Add some butter to a skillet, and once melted, spoon in some of the batter. Cook until bubbles start to form on the pancake, flip, and cook for a few minutes more.

3. Continue until the batter is used.

4. Serve with some sugar-free syrup and butter.

Keto Coffee

This recipe makes 1 serving and contains 284 calories; 24 grams fat; 16 grams protein; 0 grams net carbohydrates per serving

What You Need

- Vanilla, .25 tsp.

- Coconut oil, 1 tbsp.

- Butter, 1 tbsp.

- Brewed coffee, 1 c

What to Do

1. Add your hot coffee to a blender along with all of the other ingredients. Blend until mixed and frothy. Enjoy.

Lemon Smoothie

This recipe makes 1 serving, and contains 503 calories; 45 grams fat; 29 grams protein; 11 grams net carbohydrates per serving

What You Need

- Sweetener, 1 tsp.

- Coconut oil, 1 tbsp.

- Plain protein powder, 1 tsp.

- Lemon juice, .25 c

- Heavy cream, .25 c

- Unsweetened cashew milk, 1 c

What to Do

1. Simply place the ingredients in a blender and mix until it forms a smooth consistency. Divide into a glass and enjoy.

Breakfast Bake

This recipe makes 8 servings and contains 303 calories; 24 grams fat; 17 grams protein; 3 grams net carbohydrates per serving

What You Need

- Sausage, 1 lb.

- Eggs, 8

- Olive oil, 1 tbsp.

- Shredded cheddar, .5 c

- Pepper

- Salt

- Chopped fresh oregano, 1 tbsp.

- Cooked spaghetti squash, 2 c

What to Do

1. Start by placing your oven to 375. Grease a baking dish with some oil and place to the side.

2. Heat the olive oil in a large skillet.

3. Add in the sausage and brown. This will take about five minutes. Break apart as you cook. Beat the eggs, oregano, and squash together in a bowl. Season with a bit of pepper and salt.

4. Mix the sausage into the eggs and pour into the baking dish.

5. Sprinkle the cheese over the casserole and then wrap the dish with foil.

6. Slide this in the oven for 30 minutes. Take it out of the oven and remove the foil. Slide back in and cook for another 15 minutes.

7. Allow the casserole to cool for ten minutes before serving.

Green Smoothie

This recipe makes 2 servings and contains 436 calories; 36 grams fat; 28 grams protein; 6 grams net carbohydrates per serving

What You Need

- Vanilla protein powder, 1 scoop

- Coconut oil, 1 tbsp.

- Cream cheese, .75 c

- Shredded kale, .5 c

- Blueberries, .5 c

- Water, 1 c

What to Do

1. Simply place the ingredients in a blender and process until it reaches a smooth consistency.

2. Divide into two glasses and enjoy.

Avocado and Eggs

This recipe makes 4 servings and contains 324 calories; 25 grams fat; 19 grams protein; 3 grams net carbohydrates per serving

What You Need

- Halved and pitted avocado, 2

- Pepper

- Salt

- Cheddar cheese, .25 c

- Shredded cooked chicken breast, 4 oz.

- Eggs, 4

What to Do

1. Start by placing your oven to 425.

2. Hollow out the avocado halves until the holes left by the pit is about twice the size it was.

3. Lay the avocado halves in a baking dish with the cut side up.

4. Break an egg into each half and then top each with some of the chicken, cheese, and some pepper and salt.

5. Bake these for 15-20 minutes. Serve.

Berry Shake

This recipe makes 2 servings and contains 330 calories; 29 grams fat; 2 grams protein; 12 grams net carbohydrates per serving

What You Need

- Frozen strawberries, .5 c

- Frozen raspberries, .5 c

- Frozen blueberries, .5 c

- Vanilla, 1 tsp.

- Unsweetened coconut milk, 1 c

- Ice cubes

What to Do

1. Simply add everything to your blender and mix until it forms a smooth consistency.

2. Pour the shake into two glasses and serve.

Breakfast Crème

This recipe makes 1 serving, and contains 470 calories; 36 grams fat; 28 grams protein; 7 grams net carbohydrates per serving

What You Need

- Vanilla, .25 tsp.

- Cinnamon, .25

- Butter, 1 tsp.

- Ricotta, 1 c

What to Do

1. Place everything in a microwave safe bowl. Mix together and then microwave for a minute. Stir again and serve.

Chia Berry Smoothie Bowl

This recipe makes 3 servings and contains 401 calories; 39 grams fat; 3 grams protein; 9 grams net carbohydrates per serving

What You Need

- Liquid stevia, 3 drops

- Vanilla, 1 tsp.

- Chia seeds, 2 tbsp.

- MCT oil, 2 tbsp.

- Frozen mixed berries, 1 c

- Full-fat coconut milk, 1.5 c

- Optional Toppings:

- Almonds

- Shredded coconut

- Fresh berries

What to Do

1. Add all of the ingredients, except for the chia seeds, to your blender and mix until it forms a smooth consistency. Pour into a lidded container and stir in the chia seeds.

2. Allow this to refrigerate overnight. It will thicken up.

3. When you are ready to eat, top with your favorite toppings.

Goat Cheese Omelet

This recipe makes 4 servings and contains 506 calories; 43 grams fat; 24 grams protein; 4 grams net carbohydrates per serving

What You Need

- Pepper

- Salt

- Chopped scallions, .25 c

- Heavy cream, 4 tbsp.

- Goat cheese, 8 oz.

- Butter, 2 tbsp.

- Spinach, 6 c

- Dijon, 1 tsp.

- Olive oil, 2 tsp.

- Eggs, 8

What to Do

1. Add two teaspoons of oil to a skillet and add in the spinach. Cook until the spinach has wilted, about one to two minutes. Stir in the salt, pepper, and mustard.

2. Take the spinach out of the pan and place to the side.

3. Beat together the pepper, salt, cream, and eggs.

4. Add the butter to the skillet and melt.

5. Pour a quarter of the egg mixture into the skillet and allow the egg to set a bit. Spread a quarter of the spinach and goat cheese over the egg.

6. Cook for a few more minutes, flip, and then fold the omelet in half once the egg is completely set.

7. Continue with the rest of the eggs, making a total of four omelets.

8. Garnish the omelets with scallions.

Blueberry Muffin

This recipe makes 15 servings and contains 147 calories; 13 grams fat; 5 grams protein; 3 grams net carbohydrates per serving

What You Need

- Melted butter, 2 tbsp.

- Fresh blueberries, 4 oz.

- Eggs, 2

- Salt, .5 tsp.

- Sour cream, 1 c

- Erythritol, .25 c

- Baking soda, .5 tsp.

- Almond flour, 2 c

What to Do

1. Start by placing your oven to 350. Like a cupcake tin with paper liners, or use silicone molds.

2. Whisk together the almond flour, baking soda, and erythritol together.

3. Beat the eggs lightly and mix in the sour cream and butter. Make sure it is completely combined.

4. Pour the sour cream mixture into the almond flour mixture. Stir until completely mixed. Fold in the blueberries.

5. Divide the batter between the prepared cupcake tin holes, filling them halfway full.

6. Bake the muffins for 20 minutes. They should be golden.

7. Allow the cupcakes to cool slightly. Serve warm with a bit of butter.

Cinnamon Chia Pudding

This recipe makes 1 serving, and contains 384 calories; 24 grams fat; 16 grams protein; 28 grams net carbohydrates per serving

What You Need

- Liquid stevia, 8 drops

- Peanut butter, 1 tbsp.

- Cinnamon, .5 tsp.

- Unsweetened almond milk, 1 c

- Chia seeds, 1 tbsp.

What to Do

1. Add everything except for the chia seeds to your blender and mix until smooth.

2. Add this to a bowl and then mix in the chia seeds. Stir everything together and let it refrigerate for at least three hours. Enjoy.

Cacao Chia Shake

This recipe makes 1 serving, and contains 533 calories; 37 grams fat; 15 grams protein; 12 grams net carbohydrates per serving

What You Need

- Ice cubes, 5

- Unsweetened almond milk, 1 c

- 80-100% dark chocolate, .5 oz.

- Chia seeds, 1 tbsp.

- Avocado, .5

What to Do

1. Stir the almond milk and chia seeds together and allow this to sit for ten minutes.

2. Now, place everything in your blender and mix until smooth.

3. Pour into a glass and top with some extra dark chocolate.

Everything Bagel

This recipe makes 12 servings and contains 25 calories; 2 grams fat; 3 grams protein; 1 gram net carbohydrates per serving

What You Need

- Everything bagel seasoning

- Full-fat cream cheese, 4 oz.

- Smoked salmon, 4 oz.

- Full-fat butter, 1 tbsp.

What to Do

1. Add the cream cheese, salmon, and butter to a bowl and mix everything together until everything is well mixed. Make sure that you don't have clumps of ingredients. You want it to be very smooth.

2. Allow this to refrigerate for 30 minutes. This will let the mixture stiffen up some so that you can work with it better.

3. Once the mixture is a little firmer, divide it into 12 portions and roll them into balls.

4. Pour the bagel seasoning in a bowl and roll the balls in the seasonings. Press the seasoning into the balls so that it sticks.

5. If you don't like the taste of salmon, you can use cooked and crumbled bacon instead.

6. Once you have the bagels made, keep them refrigerated. This will allow them to stay firmer so that you can grab one and go when you don't have time to cook in the morning.

Egg Muffin Cup

This recipe makes 1 serving, and contains 294 calories; 25 grams fat; 13 grams protein; 3 grams net carbohydrates per serving

What You Need

- Pepper

- Salt

- Egg, 1

- Grated parmesan, 3 tbsp.

- Sun-dried tomatoes, 1 tbsp. – chopped

- Butter, 1 tbsp.

- Diced veggies of choice, .33 c

What to Do

1. Place one tablespoon butter into a microwave-safe mug. Put your vegetables of choice into the bottom of the mug. Put in microwave and cook one minute on high power if veggies are precooked. If the veggies are raw, cook for three minutes.

2. Add in the spinach, cheese, and one egg. Stir well to combine everything. Sprinkle with pepper and salt, stir again. Microwave one more minute.

Latkes

This recipe makes 8 servings and contains 252 calories; 21 grams fat; 5 grams protein; 4 grams net carbohydrates per serving

What You Need

- Coconut oil, 4 tbsp.

- Pepper

- Marjoram, 2 tsp.

- Psyllium husk powder, 1 tbsp.

- Flax meal, .25 c

- Egg, 1

- Sliced onion, 1 small

- Salt

- Rutabaga, 1 medium

What to Do

1. Wash and peel the rutabaga. Use a spiralizer to make noodles. A julienne peeler will also work if you don't have a spiralizer. Put the rutabaga into a colander with half a teaspoon of salt and let sit for 20 minutes.

2. Let all the moisture drain from the rutabaga. If there is any moisture left, use paper towels to blot the remaining moisture.

3. Place the onion and rutabaga into a bowl along with marjoram, psyllium powder, flax meal, and egg. Sprinkle with pepper and salt and mix well.

4. Place a skillet on medium heat and melt the coconut oil. Place spoonfuls of the mixture into the skillet to make about four latkes at one time. Flatten each with a spatula. Cook ten minutes per side until browned well.

5. Add more coconut as needed until all mixture is used up. Once everything is cooked, enjoy.

Mushroom Frittata

This recipe makes 6 servings and contains 316 calories; 27 grams fat; 16 grams protein; 1 gram net carbohydrates per serving

What You Need

- Pepper

- Salt

- Crumbled goat cheese, .5 c

- Eggs, 10

- Sliced bacon, 6

- Shredded spinach, 1 c

- Sliced mushrooms, 1 c

- Olive oil, 2 tbsp.

What to Do

1. You need to warm your oven to 350.

2. Cook the bacon in a large skillet. When crisp, take out and drain.

3. In the same skillet, add the oil and heat.

4. Add mushrooms and sauté until browned.

5. When the bacon is cool enough, crumble and add to the skillet along with the spinach until spinach is wilted.

6. Crack eggs into a bowl and beat slightly. Pour into skillet. Lift the edges of the eggs, so the uncooked eggs flow underneath for about four minutes.

7. Sprinkle top with goat cheese and season with pepper and salt.

8. Place into the oven and bake 15 minutes.

9. Take out of the oven and allow to stand for five minutes.

10. Cut into six wedges and enjoy.

Artichoke and Bacon Omelet

This recipe makes 4 servings and contains 435 calories; 39 grams fat; 17 grams protein; 3 grams net carbohydrates per serving

What You Need

- Pepper

- Salt

- Chopped artichoke hearts, .5 c

- Chopped onion, .25 c

- Olive oil, 1 tbsp.

- Sliced bacon, 8

- Heavy cream, 2 tbsp.

- Eggs, 6

What to Do

1. Place a skillet on medium heat and cook bacon. When bacon is crisp, take out, and drain. Once you can handle the bacon, crumble.

2. Add into a bowl along with heavy cream and eggs. Whisk until well blended.

3. In the same pan, add the oil and onion. Cook until softened.

4. Pour eggs into skillet. Cook, lifting edges of egg to allow uncooked portions to flow under. Do this for about two minutes.

5. Sprinkle artichoke hearts on top and gently turn the omelet over. Cook for another four minutes until the egg is set. Flip over one more time, so artichokes are on top.

6. Take off heat, slice into quarters, season with pepper and salt. Put onto plates and enjoy.

Caprese Omelet

This recipe makes 2 servings and contains 258 calories; 43 grams fat; 33 grams protein; 4 grams net carbohydrates per serving

What You Need

- Shredded mozzarella, 5 oz.

- Chopped basil, 1 tbsp.

- Halved cherry tomatoes, 3 oz.

- Pepper

- Olive oil, 2 tbsp.

- Salt

- Eggs, 6

What to Do

1. Break eggs into a bowl, sprinkle with pepper and salt. Whisk well to combine. Add in the basil. Stir well.

2. Place a skillet on top of the stove and heat on medium. Add tomatoes and fry for some time. Take the tomatoes out of the skillet. Pour the eggs into the skillet and add the tomatoes to the top. Let cook until eggs are slightly firm. Add cheese to the top.

3. Turn down the heat and cook until eggs are totally set. Take out of the pan and serve.

Lunch

Chicken Wraps

This recipe makes 4 servings and contains 264 calories; 20 grams fat; 12 grams protein; 6 grams net carbohydrates per serving

What You Need

- Chopped avocado, .5
- Chopped walnuts, .25 c
- Large lettuce leaves, 8
- Pepper
- Salt
- Chopped cooked chicken breast, 6 oz.
- Chopped fresh thyme, 2 tsp.
- Lemon juice, 1 tsp.
- Mayonnaise, .33 c

What to Do

1. Mix the thyme, lemon juice, mayonnaise, and avocado together.
2. Mix the chicken into the mixture along with some pepper and salt.
3. Divide the chicken mixture between the lettuce leaves and top with some walnuts.
4. Each person gets two wraps.

Grilled Salmon and Asparagus

This recipe makes 4 servings and contains 607 calories; 26 grams fat; 82 grams protein; 3 grams net carbohydrates per serving

What You Need

- Lemon juice, .5 tsp.

- Salmon, 4 fillets

- Garlic salt, 1 tsp.

- Pepper, .5 tsp.

- Crushed garlic, 4 cloves

- Asparagus, 1 lb.

- Basil, 2 tbsp.

- Softened butter, .25 c

What to Do

1. Add the butter to a small pot, melt, and add in the garlic. Cook this for about two minutes and then discard the garlic.

2. Add two tablespoons of butter onto the salmon and rub all over the fillets, making sure you coat both sides.

3. Lay the salmon onto a preheated grill and cook for four minutes.

4. After the first side is cooked, lay the asparagus on the grill and flip the salmon. Cook everything for another four minutes. The salmon is cooked through with it flakes easily with a fork.

5. To serve, add the rest of the butter, pepper, garlic salt, and lemon juice onto the fish.

Chicken Bacon Burger

This recipe makes 6 servings and contains 374 calories; 33 grams fat; 18 grams protein; 1 gram net carbohydrates per serving

What You Need

- Sliced avocado

- Large lettuce leaves, 6

- Coconut oil, 2 tbsp.

- Pepper

- Salt

- Chopped basil, 1 tsp.

- Ground almonds, .25 c

- Chopped bacon, 8 slices

- Ground chicken, 1 lb.

What to Do

1. Start by placing your oven to 350. Line a baking sheet with some parchment.

2. Mix together the pepper, salt, basil, almonds, bacon, and chicken.

3. Form the meat mixture into six patties.

4. Add the coconut oil to a skillet. Add the patties to the pan and sear on both sides, about three minutes on both sides.

5. Lay the patties on the baking sheet, cook them for 15 minutes, or cook until they are cooked through.

6. Serve the burgers on a lettuce leaf and topped with some avocado.

Bolognese Zoodles

This recipe makes 4 servings and contains 565 calories; 38 grams fat; 46 grams protein; 5 grams net carbohydrates per serving

What You Need

- Parmesan, .25 c
- Water, .25 c
- Crushed tomatoes, 1 can
- Oregano, 1 tsp.
- Pepper, .25 tsp.
- Salt, 1 tsp.
- Tomato paste, 2 tbsp.
- Butter, 3 tbsp.
- Basil, 1 tsp.
- Ground beef, 1.5 lbs.
- Minced garlic, 3 cloves
- Chopped celery, 1 stalk
- Chopped small onion
- Spiralized zucchini, 4

What to Do

1. Spiralize the zucchinis and lay them out on a paper towel.
2. Melt the butter in a pan and cook the onion and celery. Cook until the onions become translucent, around three minutes.
3. Mix in the garlic and sauté everything together until fragrant.
4. Mix the ground beef and cook until browned.

5. Mix in the water, pepper, salt, oregano, basil, crushed tomatoes, and tomato paste. Allow this to come up to a boil.

6. Turn the heat down and cook for about ten to 12 minutes. Everything should thicken up and be well combined.

7. Mix in the zoodles and allow the mixture to cook for four to five minutes.

8. Top with parmesan and enjoy.

Zesty Tilapia

This recipe makes 4 servings and contains 173 calories; 7 grams fat; 23 grams protein; 2 grams net carbohydrates per serving

What You Need

- Chopped parsley, 2 tsp.

- Pepper

- Minced garlic, 2 cloves

- Salt

- Juice of a lemon

- Lime juice, 1 tbsp.

- Melted butter, 2 tbsp.

- Tilapia, 4 fillets

What to Do

1. Clean and dry the tilapia.

2. Place your oven to 375.

3. Combine the pepper, salt, parsley, garlic, butter, lemon juice, and lime juice together.

4. Lay the tilapia in a baking dish and cover with the sauce. Bake the fish for 30 minutes. It should flake easily with a fork when done.

5. Serve the fish with steamed asparagus or a salad.

Avocado Pesto Zoodles

This recipe makes 4 servings and contains 526 calories; 49 grams fat; 12 grams protein; 6 grams net carbohydrates per serving

What You Need

Pesto

- Olive oil, 2 tbsp.

- Salt, 1 tsp.

- Pine nuts, .25 c

- Garlic, 3 cloves

- Fresh basil, 1 c

- Lemon juice, 1 tbsp.

- Avocados, 2

Pasta

- Parmesan, .5 c

- Bacon, 6 slices

- Olive oil, 1 tbsp.

- Spiralized zucchini, 4

What to Do

1. Start by spiralizing your zucchini and place them on paper towels to drain.

2. Add the salt, lemon juice, pine nuts, garlic, basil leaves, and avocados to your food processor. Mix for about 20-30 seconds. Add in the olive oil and mix until it creates a creamy sauce.

3. Cook your bacon in a skillet until it is crispy. Lay the bacon on paper towels to dry. Once the bacon is cool enough to handle, crumble and set to the side.

4. Add a tablespoon of oil to a pan. Cook the zoodles and toss them in the oil. Cook them for about two minutes or until tender.

5. Add the zoodles to a bowl and pour in the pesto sauce. Toss everything together and top with the crumbled bacon and parmesan cheese. Enjoy.

Roasted Chicken with Veggies

This recipe makes 6 servings and contains 407 calories; 28 grams fat; 23 grams protein; 11 grams net carbohydrates per serving

What You Need

- Pepper, 1 tsp.

- Rosemary, 1 tsp.

- Minced garlic, 3 cloves

- Chopped celery, 4 stalks

- Salt, 1 tsp.

- Chopped carrots, 2 small

- Medium onion sliced into wedges

- Olive oil, 3 tbsp.

- Bone-in, skin-on chicken thighs, 6

What to Do

1. Start by placing your oven to 400.

2. Pour the oil into a large bowl and add in the pepper, rosemary, salt, garlic, celery, carrot, and onion. Toss everything together.

3. Grease a baking dish and spread the veggies in the bottom.

4. Rub the chicken thighs with pepper and salt and lay on top of the veggies.

5. Cook everything until the veggies are tender and the chicken is cooked and browned. This should take about 35-40 minutes.

6. Allow the chicken to rest for five minutes before serving.

Shrimp Scampi with Zoodles

This recipe makes 4 servings and contains 162 calories; 7 grams fat; 18 grams protein; 5 grams net carbohydrates per serving

What You Need

- Parsley – garnish

- Parmesan, 2 tbsp.

- Spiralized zucchini, 4

- Juice of a lemon

- Chicken stock, .25 c

- Red pepper flakes, .5 tsp.

- Minced garlic, 2 cloves

- Cleaned medium shrimp, 1 lb.

- Butter, 2 tbsp.

What to Do

1. Melt the butter in a skillet. Add in the red pepper flakes and garlic. Cook everything for a minute, constantly stirring.

2. Add in the shrimp and cook for around three minutes.

3. Mix in the lemon juice and chicken stock.

4. Mix the zoodles into the mixture and cook, occasionally stirring, for around two more minutes.

5. Sprinkle with some pepper and salt.

6. Serve the shrimp scampi with some parsley and parmesan.

Taco Rolls

This recipe makes 4 servings and contains 583 calories; 40 grams fat; 48 grams protein; 3 grams net carbohydrates per serving

What You Need

- Chopped cilantro

- Tomato sauce, 1 can

- Onion powder, .5 tsp.

- Cayenne, .25 tsp.

- Cumin, .5 tsp.

- Garlic salt, .5 tsp.

- Chopped avocado, .5

- Chopped tomatoes, 25 c

- Ground beef, 1 lb.

- Taco sauce, 2 tsp.

- Cheddar cheese, 2.5 c

What to Do

1. Start by heating your oven to 400.

2. Heat a large pan and add in the beef. Cook until browned. This will take around five to seven minutes.

3. Season with some cumin, garlic salt, and onion powder.

4. Add in the tomato sauce and stir everything together so that the meat is coated. Simmer until the mixture has thickened. This will take about five minutes.

5. Lay some parchment paper on a baking sheet and spritz with cooking spray.

6. Cover the baking sheet with cheddar cheese.

7. Bake this for about 15 minutes. The cheese should be melted and bubbly but not burnt.

8. Take out of the oven and top with the taco meat. Bake for six to eight minutes more.

9. Take this out of the oven and carefully hold the sides of the parchment to remove from the baking sheet.

10. Top with cilantro, avocados, and tomatoes.

11. With a pizza cutter, slice it from top to bottom into four slices.

12. Carefully roll them up to make the taco rolls. Serve with a salad.

Fajita Bowl

This recipe makes 4 servings and contains 402 calories; 22 grams fat; 33 grams protein; 13 grams net carbohydrates per serving

What You Need

Fajita Seasoning

- Cumin, .25 tsp.

- Oregano, 1 tsp.

- Garlic powder, .25 tsp.

- Salt, .5 tsp.

- Chili powder, .5 tsp.

- Paprika, .5 tsp.

Fajitas

- Chopped cilantro, .5 c

- Sour cream, 8 oz.

- Jalapenos, .5 c

- Cherry tomatoes, 1 c

- Cubed avocado, 1 c

- Lettuce, 2 c

- Juice of ½ lime

- Sliced yellow bell pepper

- Chicken broth, .25 c

- Olive oil, 2 tbsp.

- Sliced medium onion

- Sliced red bell pepper

What to Do

1. Mix all of the fajita seasoning ingredients together.

2. Add two tablespoons of oil to a skillet and heat. Once hot, mix in the chicken and cook for five to seven minutes, or until cooked and golden.

3. Mix in the bell peppers, onion, and fajita seasoning. Let this cook for another four to five minutes, or until everything is tender.

4. Mix in the chicken brother and lime juice and let it start to boil. Turn the heat down, and cook for ten minutes.

5. Place lettuce in a serving bowl and add in the fajita meat and veggies, avocado, tomatoes, jalapenos, sour cream, and then cilantro. Enjoy.

Portobello Pizza

This recipe makes 4 servings and contains 251 calories; 20 grams fat; 14 grams protein; 4 grams net carbohydrates per serving

What You Need

- Shredded mozzarella, 1 c
- Chopped basil, 2 tsp.
- Sliced tomato, 1
- Minced garlic, 1 tsp.
- Olive oil, .25 c
- Portobello mushrooms, 4 large

What to Do

1. You need to warm your oven to broil.
2. Place aluminum foil onto a baking sheet. Grease the mushrooms with olive oil gently so you don't break them.
3. Put the mushrooms onto the baking sheet with the gill side down.
4. Place into the oven for two minutes.
5. Turn them over and broil for one more minute.
6. Remove from oven and evenly spread the garlic over each.
7. Top with a slice of tomato, a sprinkle of basil, and top with cheese.
8. Broil the mushrooms once more until cheese is bubbly and melted.

Carbonara

This recipe makes 4 servings and contains 453 calories; 80 grams fat; 25 grams protein; 9 grams net carbohydrates per serving

What You Need

- Chopped parsley

- Pepper

- Salt

- Egg yolks, 4

- Heavy whipping cream, 1.25 c

- Mayonnaise, .25 c

- Butter, 1 tbsp.

- Zucchini, 2

- Sliced bacon, 8

What to Do

1. Place the cream in a pot and allow it to boil. Turn the heat down and continue cooking for a few minutes until reduced by a fourth.

2. Cook the bacon until crisp. Keep the fat to be used later.

3. Add the mayonnaise to the cream and season with pepper and salt. Let this cook until warmed through.

4. Use a spiralizer to turn the zucchini into noodles. You could also make strips with a vegetable peeler.

5. Put the "zoodles" into the cream sauce. Divide these out into four bowls and top with parmesan, bacon, parsley, and the egg yolks. Toss to combine.

6. Drizzle with bacon grease and enjoy.

Pizza

This recipe makes 2 servings and contains 459 calories; 90 grams fat; 55 grams protein; 8 grams net carbohydrates per serving

What You Need

- Oregano, 1 tsp.

- Shredded cheddar, 5 oz.

- Olives

- Eggs, 4

- Pepperoni, 1.5 oz.

- Tomato paste, 3 tbsp.

- Shredded cheddar, 6 oz.

What to Do

1. You need to warm your oven to 400.

2. Crack the eggs in a bowl and add in six ounces of cheese. Stir until they are well combined.

3. Place parchment paper onto a baking sheet and spread the cheese batter into a thin crust. You could make two round crusts if you wanted to. Bake for 15 minutes. Take out of the oven and allow to cool.

4. Raise the oven temp to 450.

5. Spread the tomato paste on top of the crust and sprinkle with oregano. Add the remaining cheese, pepperoni, and olives.

6. Bake again for ten minutes. Serve with a salad.

Thai Zoodles

This recipe makes 2 servings and contains 644 calories; 39 grams fat; 47 grams protein; 12 grams net carbohydrates per serving

What You Need

Zoodles

- Chopped cilantro, .25 c
- Crushed peanuts, .33 c
- Bean sprouts, 1 c
- Coconut oil, 1.5 tbsp.
- Chopped green onion, .5 c
- Eggs, 2
- Shrimp, 7 oz.
- Spiralized zucchini, 2
- Lime wedges

Dressing

- Juice of a lime
- Soy sauce, 3 tbsp.
- Liquid stevia, 7 drops
- Fish sauce, 1 tbsp.
- Water, .25 c
- Peanut butter, 2 tbsp.

What to Do

1. Start by spiralizing the zucchini and set the zoodles on some paper towels to drain.

2. Mix all of the dressing ingredients together.

3. Add in ½ tablespoon of coconut oil to a large skillet, and scramble the eggs and then set them to the side.

4. Mix in the shrimp to the same pan and cook the shrimp for about three minutes or until it is pink and cooked through. Set the shrimp to the side.

5. Add a tablespoon of coconut oil into the pan and mix in the zoodles. Cook them until tender, two to three minutes.

6. Add in the cooked shrimp, scrambled eggs, and green onions.

7. Pour in the sauce and cook for another minute. Mix in the bean sprouts.

8. Serve the Pad Thai topped with a lime wedge, cilantro, and crushed peanuts.

Ricotta and Spinach Gnocchi

This recipe makes 4 servings and contains 125 calories; 8 grams fat; 6 grams protein; 4 grams net carbohydrates per serving

What You Need

- Butter, 2 tbsp.

- Water, 2.5 c

- Almond flour, just encase

- Pepper

- Salt

- Egg

- Nutmeg, .25 tsp.

- Ricotta, 1 c

- Chopped frozen spinach, 3 c

What to Do

1. Place the spinach on a paper towel or cheesecloth and squeeze the excess liquid from it. Place it in a bowl.

2. Add pepper, salt, nutmeg, egg, half of the parmesan, and the ricotta cheese into the same bowl. Mix all of the ingredients together so that they are all well combined.

3. Allow a large pot to come to a boil. Scoop out tablespoon size of the spinach mixture and roll into a cylinder shape. For a traditional gnocchi look, roll a fork across it to create lines. Add this first gnocchi to the boiling water. If the gnocchi breaks apart, mix in some almond flour to the rest of your mixture. Repeat this until the gnocchi holds together in the water.

4. Once the gnocchi holds together, form the rest of the spinach mixture into the gnocchi rounds and cook them in the boiling water. Once they rise to the top of the water, they are done. This will take about two minutes. Take the gnocchi out with a perforated spoon.

5. Melt the butter and serve the gnocchi with the melted butter over the top. Sprinkle on some parmesan cheese and serve with a salad.

Dinner

Turkey Meatloaf

This recipe makes 6 servings and contains 216 calories; 19 grams fat; 15 grams protein; 1 gram net carbohydrates per serving

What You Need

- Pepper

- Salt

- Chopped parsley, 1 tbsp.

- Parmesan, .25 c

- Heavy cream, .33 c

- Ground turkey, 1.5 lbs.

- Chopped onion, .5

- Olive oil, 1 tbsp.

What to Do

1. Start by placing your oven to 450.

2. Pour the olive oil into a skillet and cook the onion until tender, about four minutes.

3. Place the onion in a bowl and stir in the pepper, parsley, salt, parmesan, heavy cream, and turkey. Make sure everything is very well combined. Using your hands works better than a spoon to make sure everything is well combined.

4. Press the meat into a loaf pan.

5. Bake for 30 minutes.

6. Allow the meatloaf to rest for ten before serving.

Haddock

This recipe makes 4 servings and contains 299 calories; 24 grams fat; 20 grams protein; 1 gram net carbohydrates per serving

What You Need

- Melted coconut oil, 2 tbsp.

- Ground hazelnuts, .25 c

- Shredded unsweetened coconut, 1 c

- Pepper

- Salt

- Boneless haddock 4 5-oz. fillets

What to Do

1. Start by placing your oven to 400. Place parchment paper on a baking sheet.

2. Dry off the fillets with a paper towel, and then sprinkle them with pepper and salt on both sides.

3. Mix the hazelnuts and shredded coconut together.

4. Brush the fillets with coconut oil, and then press the coconut mixture into the fish.

5. Bake the fish for 12 minutes. It should flake apart easily. Serve.

Zucchini Gratin

This recipe makes 4 servings and contains 371 calories; 33 grams fat; 13 grams protein; 4 grams net carbohydrates per serving

What You Need

- Pepper

- Salt

- Shredded cheese, 1.5 c

- Heavy cream, 1 c

- Sliced yellow squash, 2

- Sliced zucchini, 2

- Minced garlic, 2 cloves

- Diced small onion

- Butter, 2 tbsp.

What to Do

1. Start by placing your oven to 350.

2. Melt the butter in a skillet. Mix in the onions and cook until they become translucent.

3. Mix in the garlic and sauté everything for a minute.

4. Mix in the heavy cream and a cup of the cheese. Make sure you stir quickly and make sure everything is well mixed, and the cheese has melted.

5. Let the sauce simmer until it has thickened.

6. Meanwhile, grease a baking dish with some cooking spray.

7. Lay the squash and zucchini in the baking dish. Pour the cheese sauce on the veggies and top with the remaining shredded cheese.

8. Bake this for 30 minutes, or until it has thickened and the top has browned.

9. Serve.

Cauliflower Mac and Cheese

This recipe makes 4 servings and contains 434 calories; 39 grams fat; 15 grams protein; 5 grams net carbohydrates per serving

What You Need

- Pepper

- Salt

- Garlic powder, .5 tsp.

- Dijon, 1 tsp.

- Shredded cheddar, 1 ½ c – divided

- Cubed cream cheese, 4 oz.

- Heavy cream, .5 c

- Olive oil, 2 tsp.

- Butter, 2 tbsp.

- Bacon, 2 slices

- Cauliflower, 1 head – cut into florets

What to Do

4. Start by setting your oven to 425 and heat the oil in a pan.

5. Place the cauliflower and bacon in the pan and cook for five minutes.

6. Pour this into a casserole dish and place this to the side.

7. In a pot, add a cup of cheddar, heavy cream, Dijon, and butter. Cook, stirring until everything is melted and combined. Whisk the cream cheese into the mixture until melted and smooth. Season with garlic powder, pepper, and salt.

8. Pour the cheese over the cauliflower and mix everything together. Sprinkle on the remaining cheese and bake for 15 minutes. The top should be browned. Enjoy.

Lettuce Wrap Cheeseburger

This recipe makes 1 serving, and contains 601 calories; 51 grams fat; 26 grams protein; 5 grams net carbohydrates per serving

What You Need

- Mayonnaise, 1 tsp.

- Oregano, 1 tsp.

- Salt, .5 tsp.

- Onion, 3 rings

- Pepper, .25 tsp.

- Lettuce leaves

- Slice cheese

- Ground beef, 5 oz.

What to Do

1. Season the meat with oregano, pepper, and salt. Form the meat into a patty.

2. Grill the burger for four to five minutes on both sides or until it is cooked to your liking.

3. Once the burger is cooked, take it off the grill and top with a slice of cheese and lay it on top of the lettuce leaf.

4. Top with the onion and mayonnaise. Wrap the lettuce around and enjoy.

Pork Loin with Mustard Sauce

This recipe makes 8 servings and contains 368 calories; 29 grams fat; 25 grams protein; 2 grams net carbohydrates per serving

What You Need

- Grainy mustard, 3 tbsp.

- Heavy cream, 1.5 c

- Olive oil, 3 tbsp.

- Pepper

- Salt

- Boneless pork loin roast, 2 lb.

What to Do

1. Start by placing your oven to 375.

2. Rub the pork loin with pepper and salt.

3. Heat the oil in a large skillet. Place the roast in the hot pan and sear on all sides. Lay in a baking dish.

4. Finish cooking the roast in the oven for an hour.

5. When about 15 minutes remain on the roasting time, add the mustard and heavy cream to a pot. Stir together and allow it to start boiling. Lower to a simmer and allow the mixture to continue to simmer until it has thickened up, about five minutes. Set it off the heat.

6. Once the pork is cooked to your liking, allow it to cool for ten minutes before slicing. Serve with a drizzle of mustard sauce.

Lamb with Sun-Dried Tomatoes

This recipe makes 8 servings and contains 352 calories; 29 grams fat; 17 grams protein; 3 grams net carbohydrates per serving

What You Need

Lamb

- Olive oil, 2 tbsp.

- Pepper

- Salt

- Boneless lamb leg, 2 lb.

Pesto

- Minced garlic, 2 tsp.

- Chopped basil, 2 tbsp.

- EVOO, 2 tbsp.

- Pine nuts, .25 c

- Sun-dried tomatoes, 1 c

What to Do

1. **For the pesto** – Place the pest ingredients in your food processor and mix until the sauce becomes smooth. Set aside.

2. **For the lamb** – begin by placing your oven to 400.

3. Rub the leg of lamb with pepper and salt.

4. Add the oil to an ovenproof skillet and heat. Sear the lamb on all sides until it has browned up.

5. Rub the leg of lamb with the pesto sauce. Roast for an hour, or until the lamb has reached your desired doneness.

6. Allow the lamb to sit for ten minutes before slicing and serving.

Thai Lettuce Wrap

This recipe makes 6 servings and contains 286 calories; 15 grams fat; 22 grams protein; 13 grams net carbohydrates per serving

What You Need

- Pepper

- Salt

- Chopped peanuts, .25 c

- Chopped cilantro, .25 c

- Chopped green onions, 3

- Chopped large onion

- Minced garlic, 3 cloves

- Diced chicken breasts, 1 lb.

- Olive oil, 1 tbsp.

- Large head iceberg

Sauce

- Ginger, .25 tsp.

- Peanut butter, 1 tbsp.

- Chili sauce, .25 c

- Soy sauce, 1 tbsp.

- Juice of ½ lime

- Fish sauce, 2 tsp.

What to Do

1. Heat the oil in a large skillet.

2. Add in the onion, stir often, cooking until soft. This will take about four minutes.

3. Stir in the garlic, cooking for another minute.

4. Mix in the chicken and turn the heat up. Cook for about three minutes, or until the chicken is almost cooked.

5. Add the sauce ingredients to a bowl and mix them together.

6. Pour the sauce into the skillet with the chicken and stir everything to coat. Continue the cook until the chicken is cooked all the way through. This will take about five minutes more.

7. Mix in the peanuts, cilantro, and green onions. Toss everything together. Taste and adjust any seasonings that you need to.

8. Spoon the chicken into the lettuce leaves and serve.

Cheeseburger

This recipe makes 4 servings and contains 850 calories; 67 grams fat; 49 grams protein; 7 grams net carbohydrates per serving

What You Need

- Pepper, .5 tsp.

- Salt, 1 tsp.

- Peanut butter, 4 tbsp.

- Bacon, 20 slices

- Onion powder, 1 tsp.

- Cheddar cheese, 2 oz.

- Garlic powder, 1 tsp.

- Ground beef, 1 lb.

What to Do

1. Using your hands, mix together the ground beef and the seasonings. Form the meat into four patties.

2. Grill the burgers until they are almost done. They will cook more later on, so you don't want them to become tough.

3. Once the burgers are done, spread each with a tablespoon of peanut butter and top with a sprinkle of cheese.

4. Wrap five slices of bacon around each burger and lay them on a cookie sheet.

5. Cook the burgers for 20 minutes at 400. Cook until the bacon is done to your liking.

6. Serve your burger with onion, lettuce, and any other desired toppings.

Tri-Tip

This recipe makes 4 servings and contains 693 calories; 44 grams fat; 68 grams protein; 0 gram net carbohydrates per serving

What You Need

- Salt, .5 tbsp.

- Pepper, 1 tsp.

- Minced garlic clove

- Olive oil, 3 tbsp.

- Tri-tip steak, 2 lbs.

What to Do

1. Mix together the pepper, salt, oil, and garlic. Rub the steak with the marinade and refrigerate it for a couple of hours.

2. Heat a skillet and place in the steak. Cook the steak for five minutes on both sides.

3. Slice the steak and serve with a salad.

Sausage Casserole

This recipe makes 4 servings and contains 332 calories; 26 grams fat; 18 grams protein; 4 grams net carbohydrates per serving

What You Need

- Shredded cheddar, 1 c
- Ground sage, 1 tsp.
- Mayonnaise, 2 tsp.
- Eggs, 3
- Diced zucchini, 2
- Dijon, 1 tsp.
- Diced onion, .5 c
- Pork sausage, .5 lb.

What to Do

1. Start by placing your oven to 375.
2. Grease a baking dish with some nonstick spray.
3. Heat a large pan and add in the sausage. Cook until the sausage has browned up, about two minutes.
4. Mix in the onion and zucchini. Cook for another four to five minutes or until the veggies become tender.
5. Spoon this into the greased baking dish.
6. Stir together ½ cup of cheese, the sage, mustard, mayonnaise, and eggs.
7. Pour this over the sausage mixture.
8. Top with the rest of the cheese and bake for 25 minutes. Enjoy.

Sausage Crust Pizza

This recipe makes 4 servings and contains 357 calories; 21 grams fat; 31 grams protein; 12 grams net carbohydrates per serving

What You Need

- Italian seasoning, 1 tsp.

- Onion powder, 1 tsp.

- Tomato paste, 1 tbsp.

- Sliced ham, 2 oz.

- Garlic powder, 1 tsp.

- Diced red bell pepper

- Diced and sautéed small onion

- Mozzarella cheese, 3 oz.

- Sautéed mushrooms, 2 oz.

- Sausage, 1 lb.

What to Do

1. Start by placing your oven to 350.

2. Mash the sausage into the bottom and sides of a medium cake pan. Bake this for 10-15 minutes.

3. Take the crust out and drain off any grease that has accumulated.

4. Combine the Italian seasoning, onion powder, garlic powder, and tomato paste. Spread this over the crust.

5. Top with the mushrooms, bell pepper, ham, and onions.

6. Sprinkle the top with the mozzarella.

7. Cook the pizza until the cheese is melted and bubbly, about 12-15 minutes.

Garlic Parmesan Salmon

This recipe makes 2 servings and contains 480 calories; 33 grams fat; 35 grams protein; 8 grams net carbohydrates per serving

What You Need

- Pepper

- Salt

- Chopped parsley, 1 bunch

- Heavy cream, .25 c

- Parmesan, .5 c

- Minced garlic, 3 cloves

- Butter, 2 tbsp.

- Salmon, 2 9-oz. fillets

What to Do

1. Start by placing your oven to 350.

2. Line a baking sheet with parchment.

3. Lay the salmon on the baking sheet and sprinkle with some pepper and salt, and set to the side.

4. Melt the butter in a skillet. Mix in the garlic and sauté until softened. Turn the heat down and mix in the parmesan and heavy cream. Mix everything together until melted.

5. Pour this over the salmon.

6. Bake for 15-20 minutes. Sprinkle on a little more salt and top with some parsley. Serve with a salad.

Coconut Lime Skirt Steak

This recipe makes 3 servings and contains 787 calories; 48 grams fat; 89 grams protein; 2 grams net carbohydrates per serving

What You Need

- Salt, 1 tsp.

- Grated ginger, 1 tbsp.

- Lime juice, 2 tbsp.

- Melted coconut oil, .5 c

- Minced garlic, 1 tbsp.

- Skirt steak, 2 lbs.

What to Do

1. Combine the salt, ginger, garlic, lime juice, and melted coconut oil together.

2. Put the steak in a bag and add in the marinade. Allow this to sit for at least 30 minutes. Make sure you don't skip this.

3. Grill the steak for at least four minutes on each side. You can cook it longer to reach your desired level of doneness. Slice and serve.

Creamy Butter Chicken

This recipe makes 6 servings and contains 319 calories; 20 grams fat; 26 grams protein; 5 grams net carbohydrates per serving

What You Need

For Serving

- Cooked cauliflower rice
- Chopped cilantro

Sauce

- Garam masala, .5 tbsp.
- Heavy cream, .5 c
- Cumin, 1 tsp.
- Chili powder, 1 tsp.
- Crushed tomatoes, small can
- Minced garlic, 2 tsp.
- Tomato paste, 2 tbsp.
- Grated ginger, 2 tsp.
- Chopped onion
- Ghee, 2 tbsp.
- Chicken –
- Plain yogurt, 4 oz.
- Minced garlic, 3 cloves
- Olive oil, 1 tbsp.

- Grated ginger, 3 tsp.

- Garam masala, 2 tbsp.

Diced chicken breast, 1.5 lbs.

What to Do

1. Add the chicken and two tablespoons of garam masala, along with the yogurt, minced garlic, and grated ginger to a bowl and mix them together. Chill the chicken for at least 20 minutes.

2. For the sauce – add the tomato paste, tomatoes, garlic, ginger, and onion to a blender and combine everything until smooth. Set to the side.

3. Heat a tablespoon of oil in a large pan.

4. Add the chicken to the pan and sauté for four to five minutes, or until it turns golden.

5. Add the sauce into the chicken and cook for another four to six minutes more.

6. Mix in the ghee and heavy cream. Turn the heat down and cook for another five minutes.

7. Serve the chicken over top of the cooked cauliflower rice and topped with cilantro.

Buffalo Chicken

This recipe makes 2 servings and contains 685 calories; 43 grams fat; 57 grams protein; 12 grams net carbohydrates per serving

What You Need

- Pepper, 2 tsp.

- Chili powder, 1 tsp.

- Garlic powder, 1 tsp.

- Eggs, 2

- Salt, 2 tsp.

- Blue cheese dip, .5 c

- Butter, 2 tbsp.

- Hot sauce, .25 c

- Paprika, 1 tsp.

- Almond flour, 2 tbsp.

- Chicken breast strips, 1 lb.

What to Do

1. Start by placing your oven to 400.

2. Line a baking sheet with parchment.

3. Mix together the pepper, salt, chili powder, paprika, and garlic powder.

4. Rub a quarter of the spice mixture onto the chicken.

5. Place the remaining seasonings in the almond flour and mix together.

6. Beat the eggs together in a separate bowl.

7. Coat the chicken tender in the egg and then dip into the almond flour. Lay the chicken on your baking sheet. Repeat this for the rest of the chicken.

8. Bake the chicken tenders for 25 minutes. They should reach 165.

9. Meanwhile, add the butter to a pot and melt. Mix in the hot sauce and combined well.

10. Once the chicken is done, drizzle the hot sauce over the chicken. You can also toss the chicken tenders in the sauce to completely cover them.

11. Serve with the blue cheese dip.

Sausage and Veggies

This recipe makes 4 servings and contains 220 calories; 12 grams fat; 15 grams protein; 10 grams net carbohydrates per serving

What You Need

- Pepper

- Salt

- Italian seasoning, .5 tsp.

- Vegetable broth, .5 c

- Baby spinach, 1 c

- Medium zucchini sliced into half-moon shapes

- Chopped yellow bell pepper

- Chopped mushrooms, 1 c

- Chopped red bell pepper

- Sliced onion

- Minced garlic, 2 cloves

- Cooked, sliced Italian chicken sausage, 12 oz.

- Olive oil, 1.5 tbsp.

What to Do

1. Heat the oil in a large pan.

2. Mix in the onion and sausage and cook until the onions have become tender.

3. Mix in the garlic, cooking everything for another minute.

4. Mix in the pepper, salt, Italian seasoning, mushrooms, bell peppers, and zucchini. Sauté everything for two minutes.

5. Pour in the broth and let the mixture come to a boil. Lower to a simmer and cook for ten minutes.

6. Mix in the spinach, cooking until wilted.

7. Serve.

Stuffed Peppers

This recipe makes 2 servings and contains 453 calories; 30 grams fat; 28 grams protein; 9 grams net carbohydrates per serving

What You Need

- Pepper

- Salt

- Shredded cheddar, .25 c

- Chopped cilantro, .25 c

- Sliced mushrooms, 8

- Minced garlic clove

- Poblano peppers halved vertically, 4

- Coconut oil, 1 tbsp.

- Chorizo sausage, .5 lb.

What to Do

1. Start by placing the oven to 375.

2. Let the peppers on a baking sheet and slide them in the oven for ten minutes.

3. Meanwhile, add the chorizo in a skillet with the coconut oil and cook for four to five minutes, or until browned.

4. Mix in the garlic, stirring until fragrant. Mix in the mushrooms.

5. After the mushrooms have browned up, mix in the cilantro and cook for three minutes more.

6. Take the peppers out of the oven and divide the chorizo mixture between them. Sprinkle the tops of the peppers with the cheddar.

7. Cook the peppers for eight minutes.

8. Serve.

Crispy Wings

This recipe makes 2 servings and contains 582 calories; 16 grams fat; 99 grams protein; 5 grams net carbohydrates per serving

What You Need

- Salt, 2 tsp.

- Chicken wings, 2 lbs.

- Baking powder, 1.5 tbsp.

What to Do

1. Set your oven to 250.

2. Get the chicken wings as dry as possible and then lay them in a plastic bag. Pour in the salt and baking powder. Shake everything together so that they are well coated.

3. Spread the chicken wings out on a baking sheet and slide them in the oven for 30 minutes.

4. Turn the temperature up to 425 and continue to cook the chicken for 20-30 minutes, or until they are completely cooked.

5. You can enjoy them as is or toss them in your favorite sauce.

Pulled Pork

This recipe makes 8 servings and contains 464 calories; 30 grams fat; 43 grams protein; 2 grams net carbohydrates per serving

What You Need

- Bay leaves, 3

- Garlic powder, 2 tsp.

- Salt, 3 tsp.

- Boneless pork shoulder, 3 lb.

- Paprika, 1 tsp.

- Chopped onion

What to Do

1. Flip your crockpot to low.

2. Combine some salt, paprika, and garlic powder.

3. Slice some lines into the surface of the pork should so that it has some areas to catch the spices. Rub the spice mixture into the pork.

4. Lay the pork and the onion into your crockpot.

5. Top with the bay leaves.

6. Place on the lid and let it cook for ten minutes.

7. Once it's cooked through, remove the bay leaves, and shred the pork.

8. Serve hot with your favorite low-carb barbecue sauce.

Dijon Chicken with Vegetables

This recipe makes 4 servings and contains 603 calories; 46 grams fat; 34 grams protein; 8 grams net carbohydrates per serving

What You Need

- Juice of lemon

- Cauliflower florets, 2 c

- Broccoli florets, 2 c

- Medium carrots cut into 4-inch pieces, 4

- Fresh thyme, 1 tbsp.

- Minced garlic clove

- Dijon, 3 tbsp. – divided

- Sliced medium onion, 3

- Olive oil, 4 tbsp. – divided

- Salt, 3 tsp. – divided

- Skin-on bone-in chicken thighs, 4

What to Do

1. Start by placing your oven to 425.

2. Mix together two teaspoons of salt, a tablespoon of garlic, two tablespoons of mustard, and two tablespoons of oil. Brush the mixture onto the chicken thighs.

3. Lay the chicken thighs with the skin side up on a baking sheet. Bake the chicken for ten minutes.

4. As the chicken is cooking, mix the rest of the salt, oil, mustard, lemon juice, and thyme. Toss in the cauliflower, broccoli, carrots, and onions. Toss everything together.

5. Lay the vegetables on a baking sheet. Once ten minutes of cooking time has passed, add the veggies to the oven and let everything cook for 25 minutes more, or until the chicken is cooked and the vegetables are tender.

6. Garnish with some extra thyme.

Indian-Style Chicken

This recipe makes 4 servings and contains 563 calories; 30 grams fat; 63 grams protein; 4 grams net carbohydrates per serving

What You Need

- Pepper

- Salt

- Steamed broccoli, 4 c

- Cumin, 1 tsp.

- Full-fat Greek yogurt, 1 c

- Chopped onion

- Turmeric, .5 tsp.

- Grated ginger, 1 tbsp.

- Olive oil, 1 tbsp.

- Cayenne, .5 tsp.

- Minced garlic, 3 cloves

- Boneless, skinless chicken breasts, 4

What to Do

1. Add the pepper, salt, turmeric, cayenne, oil, ginger, onion, yogurt, and chicken to a plastic bag and toss everything together.

2. Refrigerate the chicken for at least two hours.

3. Set your oven to 350.

4. Grease a baking sheet.

5. Take the chicken out of the bag and lay it out on the baking sheet. Cook the chicken for ten minutes.

6. Take the chicken out of the oven and flip. Cook for another ten minutes.

7. Slice the chicken and serve with the steamed broccoli.

Mexican Meatloaf

This recipe makes 8 servings and contains 372 calories; 20 grams fat; 40 grams protein; 2 grams net carbohydrates per serving

What You Need

- Chopped small onion
- Grated cheddar, 1 c
- Chili powder, 2 tsp.
- Pork rind crumbs, 1 c
- Pepper, .5 tsp.
- Cumin, 2 tsp.
- Salsa, .5 c
- Eggs, 2
- Ground beef, 2 lbs.

What to Do

1. Start by placing your oven to 350.
2. Mix together the onion, pepper, cumin, chili powder, eggs, pork rinds, and ground beef. Using your hands is the best option because you can get everything mixed together better.
3. Press half of the meatloaf mixture into a loaf pan.
4. Sprinkle half of a cup of the cheese.
5. Press the rest of the meatloaf mixture over top of the cheese.
6. Bake the meatloaf for an hour.
7. Top with the remaining cheese and bake for an additional ten minutes, or until the cheese has melted.
8. Allow the meatloaf to rest for ten minutes before slicing and serving.

Chicken Enchiladas

This recipe makes 4 servings and contains 297 calories; 16 grams fat; 32 grams protein; 3 grams net carbohydrates per serving

What You Need

- Shredded cheddar, 1 c
- Shredded Jack cheese, 1 c
- Cumin, 2 tsp.
- Chili powder, 2 tsp.
- Butter, 1 tbsp.
- Zucchinis sliced into flat sheets, 4
- Cubed medium onion
- Shredded cooked chicken, 1 lb.

Enchilada Sauce

- Pepper, 1 tsp.
- Onion powder, 1 tsp.
- Hot sauce, .5 tsp.
- Garlic powder, 1 tsp.
- Water, .5 c
- Olive oil, .25 c
- Italian seasoning, 1 tsp.
- Tomato paste, 1 can

What to Do

1. Start by placing your oven to 350.

2. Mix all of the sauce ingredients together.

3. Melt the butter in a large skillet. Sauté the onions in the butter until they are soft, about three to four minutes.

4. Mix in the cumin, chili powder, shredded chicken, and a cup of the enchilada sauce. Set to the side.

5. Lay four slices of zucchini side by side, overlapping them slightly.

6. Add a spoonful of the chicken to one end of the zucchini and roll them up. Place it in the casserole dish.

7. Continue this process until you have used the rest of the chicken and zucchini.

8. Next, pour the rest of the enchilada sauce over the rolled zucchini and then sprinkle both kinds of cheese over the top.

9. Slide them in the oven and cook for 20 to 25 minutes, or until the cheese has melted and is bubbly.

10. Serve with any of your favorite toppings like sour cream.

Halibut Butter Sauce

This recipe makes 4 servings and contains 319 calories; 26 grams fat; 22 grams protein; 2 grams net carbohydrates per serving

What You Need

- Olive oil, 2 tbsp.

- Halibut fillets, 4 5-oz. fillets

- Pepper

- Chopped parsley, 1 tsp.

- Lemon juice, 1 tbsp.

- Butter, .25 c

- Orange juice, 1 tbsp.

- Minced garlic, 2 tsp.

- Minced shallot

- Dry white wine, 3 tbsp.

What to Do

1. Pat the halibut dry so that it holds onto the seasoning. Rub the pepper and salt into the fish. Lay on a plate lined with paper towels and set to the side.

2. Place the butter in a pot and allow it to melt.

3. Add in the garlic and shallot and cook until it becomes tender. This will take around three minutes.

4. Mix in the orange juice, white wine, and lemon juice. Allow this sauce to simmer and cook until it has slightly thickened. This is going to take around two minutes.

5. Set it off the heat and mix in the parsley. Set to the side.

6. Heat a large skillet with the olive oil.

7. Fry up the fish until it is golden and cooked all the way through, flipping only once. This will take around ten minutes.

8. Serve the fish with a spoonful of the butter sauce.

Lamb Chops with Tapenade

This recipe makes 4 servings and contains 348 calories; 28 grams fat; 21 grams protein; 1 gram net carbohydrates per serving

What You Need

Tapenade

- Chopped fresh parsley, 2 tbsp.

- Kalamata olives, 1 c

- Lemon juice, 2 tsp.

- Minced garlic, 2 tsp.

- EVOO, 2 tbsp.

Lamb Chops

- French-cut lamb chips, 2 1-lb. racks

- Olive oil, 1 tbsp.

- Pepper

- Salt

What to Do

1. To make the tapenade, place the olives, lemon juice, parsley, garlic, and olive oil in a food processor and mix until it is completely pureed but still a little bit chunky.

2. Pour the tapenade into a container and keep it refrigerated until you need it.

3. To make the lamb chops, start by setting your oven to 450. Rub the pepper and the salt into the lamb.

4. Drizzle the oil into an ovenproof skillet and allow it to heat up. Lay the lamb racks in the pan and sear on all sides.

5. Sit the racks upright in the heated pan. The bones need to be interlaced. Roast the lamb in the oven until it has reached your desired level of doneness. 20 minutes will bring the lamb to about medium-rare. At the very least, it should reach 125.

6. Once the lamb is finished cooking, let it rest for ten minutes. Slice up the rack of lambs into individual chops. Each person should get four chops and top each of them with some of the tapenade you fixed earlier.

Sirloin and Butter

This recipe makes 4 servings and contains 544 calories; 44 grams fat; 35 grams protein; 0 gram net carbohydrates per serving

What You Need

- Room temperature butter, 6 tbsp.

- Pepper

- Blue cheese, 4 oz.

- Salt

- Sirloin steaks, 4 5-oz. steaks

- Olive oil, 1 tbsp.

What to Do

1. Place the butter in a blender and whip it up. This will take about two minutes.

2. Place the cheese in with the butter and pulse a few times until mixed.

3. Spoon the butter out on saran wrap and roll it up into a log that is about 1.5 inches in diameter.

4. Refrigerate the butter for at least an hour to allow it to set up.

5. Slice the butter into half-inch disks and lay them on a plate. Keep them in the refrigerator until you are ready to use them. Any leftover butter should be kept in the fridge as well, and it should last for up to a week.

6. Heat a grill or skillet. Make sure that the steak comes to room temperature before cooking.

7. Rub the salt, oil, and pepper into the steaks.

8. Cook the steaks until they are done to how you like them. Six minutes on both sides will bring it to medium. Remember, the steaks will continue to cook once you take them off the heat. Typically, it will rise five degrees during the resting period.

9. Let the steak rest for ten minutes. Serve each steak with one of the butter disks.

Noodles with Beef Stroganoff Meatballs

This recipe makes 3 servings and contains 492 calories; 39 grams fat; 19 grams protein; 14 grams net carbohydrates per serving

What You Need

- Onion powder, .5 tsp.

- Dried parsley, .5 tsp.

- Worcestershire sauce, 1 tsp.

- Almond flour, 3 tbsp.

- Pepper, .25 tsp.

- Salt, 1 tsp.

- Garlic powder, .5 tsp.

- Egg

- Ground beef, .5 tsp.

Sauce

- Butter, 2 tbsp.

- Konjac noodles, 2 servings

- Sliced mushrooms, 8 oz.

- Xanthan gum, pinch

- Sliced medium onion

- Pepper, .25 tsp.

- Minced garlic, 3 cloves

- Salt, 1 tsp.

- Beef broth, .75 c

- Sour cream, .33 c

What to Do

1. Start by placing your oven to 400. Place some parchment on a cookie sheet.

2. Add all of the meatball ingredients in a bowl and combine. Use an ice cream scoop to help you shape the meat into balls. Lay them on your cookie sheet and bake the meatballs for ten minutes.

3. As the meatballs are cooking, add the butter to a skillet and melt. Mix in the onions, cooking until translucent. Mix in the mushrooms and cook for another seven minutes. Stir in the garlic and cook until fragrant.

4. Stir in the sour cream, salt, pepper, xanthan gum, and broth. Let this mixture come up to a simmer.

5. Once the meatballs have cooked in the oven, nestle them into the sauce. Cover the skillet with a lid and let everything cook together for 20 minutes.

6. Top the konjac noodles with the meatballs and sauce.

Chicken Cordon Bleu Casserole

This recipe makes 4 servings and contains 574 calories; 34 grams fat; 59 grams protein; 3 grams net carbohydrates per serving

What You Need

- Diced onion, .25 c

- Minced garlic, 2 cloves

- Dijon, 2 tsp.

- Sliced Swiss cheese, 3 oz.

- Lemon juice, 3 tbsp.

- Sliced chicken, 1 lb.

- Melted butter, .25 c + 1 tbsp.

- Sliced ham, 3 oz.

- Salt, 1 tsp.

- Softened cream cheese, 3 oz.

What to Do

1. Start by placing your oven to 350. Spray a 9-inch square casserole dish with nonstick spray and set to the side.

2. Add a tablespoon of butter and the diced onion to a skillet and cook until the onions become translucent. This will take about five minutes. Mix in the garlic, and cook until the garlic has become fragrant.

3. Add the rest of the butter, cream cheese, Dijon, lemon juice, and salt to a blender and mix until smooth.

4. Lay the chicken in your casserole dish and then add in with the onion mixture. Lay the ham over top and then spread the sauce over everything.

5. Top the casserole with the sliced Swiss cheese. Bake the casserole for 35 minutes.

6. Once the cooking time has ended, flip the oven to broil and bake the casserole for another two minutes until the cheese has browned and everything is bubbly. Allow the casserole to rest for a few minutes before serving.

Turkey Mushroom Bake

This recipe makes 8 servings and contains 245 calories; 15 grams fat; 25 grams protein; 3 grams net carbohydrates per serving

What You Need

- Garlic powder, .25 tsp.

- Pepper

- Salt

- Grated parmesan, .5 c

- Grated cheddar cheese, 2 c

- Poultry seasoning, 1 tsp.

- Cream cheese, .5 c

- Chicken stock, .5 c

- Cooked and shredded turkey, 3 c

- Shredded cabbage, 3 c

- Beaten egg

- Sliced mushrooms, 4 c

What to Do

1. Start by placing your oven to 375.

2. Heat a skillet and add in the salt, cream cheese, cheddar cheese, poultry seasoning, garlic powder, pepper, parmesan cheese, and egg. Mix everything together and allow it to come to a simmer.

3. Mix in the turkey and cabbage and then set to the side.

4. Add the mushrooms and the turkey mixture to a casserole dish and spread across the bottom.

5. Cover with aluminum foil and cook the casserole for 35 minutes.

6. Let the casserole rest for a few minutes before serving.

Turkey Pot Pie

This recipe makes 4 servings and contains 325 calories; 23 grams fat; 21 grams protein; 6 grams net carbohydrates per serving

What You Need

- Cooking spray

- Xanthan gum, .25 tsp.

- Garlic powder, .25 tsp.

- Smoked paprika, .25 tsp.

- Shredded Monterey Jack, .5 c

- Chopped and peeled butternut squash, .5 c

- Chopped kale, .5 c

- Chopped fresh rosemary, 1 tsp.

- Pepper

- Salt

- Cooked and shredded turkey, 1 c

- Chicken stock, 2 c

Crust

- Cheddar cheese, .25 c

- Egg

- Pinch of salt

- Almond flour, 2 c

- Xanthan gum, .25 tsp.

- Butter, .25 c

What to Do

1. Start by placing your oven to 350.

2. Heat a large pot and add in the squash and turkey. Cook the two for ten minutes. Mix in the salt, kale, smoked paprika, pepper, rosemary, garlic powder, and Monterey jack cheese.

3. In a bowl, mix together the xanthan gum and stock. Pour this into the pot with everything else and mix together. Set this to the side.

4. Mix the flour and xanthan gum for the crust together. Stir the rest of the crust ingredients in until it forms a dough.

5. Roll into a ball and refrigerate for a few minutes while you get everything else ready.

6. Grease a square baking dish with cooking spray and the turkey filling into the casserole dish.

7. Take the crust out of the fridge and place it between two sheets of parchment. Roll the dough out so that it will cover the casserole dish. Lay the dough over the turkey filling and crimp down the edges to seal.

8. Bake for 35 minutes.

9. Allow the pie rest for a few minutes and serve.

Buttered Duck

This recipe makes 1 serving, and contains 547 calories; 46 grams fat; 35 grams protein; 2 grams net carbohydrates per serving

What You Need

- Fresh sage, .25 tsp.

- Kale, 1 c

- Pepper

- Salt

- Butter, 2 tbsp.

- Heavy cream, 1 tbsp.

- Medium duck breast – skin scored

What to Do

1. Place the butter on a pan. Once melted, add in the heavy cream and the sage. Cook this for two minutes.

2. In another pan, place the duck with the skin side down. Cook the duck for four minutes to brown the skin, and then flip and cook for another three minutes or until the duck is cooked through to 160.

3. Add the kale to the skillet with the butter and sage. Cook this for a minute.

4. Once the duck is cooked through, remove from the pan and slice. Place the duck on a plate and serve topped with the kale and butter sauce.

Cheesy Salmon

This recipe makes 4 servings and contains 357 calories; 28 grams fat; 24 grams protein; 2 grams net carbohydrates per serving

What You Need

- Olive oil, 1 tbsp.

- Chopped basil, 1 tsp.

- Salmon filet, skin on, 4 5 oz.

- Chopped oregano, 1 tsp.

- Minced garlic, 2 tsp.

- Room temp butter, 2 tbsp.

- Lemon juice, 2 tbsp.

- Asiago cheese, .5 c

What to Do

1. You need to warm your oven to 350.

2. Line a baking sheet with parchment.

3. Put the Asiago cheese, oregano, basil, garlic, butter, and lemon juice into a bowl. Stir together.

4. Put the salmon on the prepared baking sheet with the skin down.

5. Take the cheese mixture and divide it evenly between the salmon fillets. Spread it on the salmon with a spoon.

6. Drizzle lightly with olive oil.

7. Place in the oven for 12 minutes.

Herbed Scallops

This recipe makes 4 servings and contains 306 calories; 24 grams fat; 19 grams protein; 4 grams net carbohydrates per serving

What You Need

- Chopped thyme, 1 tsp.

- Juice of one lemon

- Minced garlic, 2 tsp.

- Chopped basil, 2 tsp.

- Butter, 8 tbsp., divided

- Pepper

- Scallops, 1 lb.

What to Do

1. Sprinkle pepper on the scallops.

2. Put a large skillet on to the top of the stove and melt the butter over medium.

3. Lay the scallops to the pan and sear on each side. This will take around two minutes. Take the scallops out of the skillet and place to the side.

4. Put the remaining butter in the skillet and add garlic. Cook until fragrant. This takes around three minutes.

5. Mix the thyme, basil and lemon juice to the garlic in the skillet. Return the scallops to the skillet.

6. Spoon the butter mixture over the scallops to coat.

Buttery Lemon Chicken

This recipe makes 4 servings and contains 294 calories; 26 grams fat; 12 grams protein; 3 grams net carbohydrates per serving

What You Need

- Juice of .5 lemon

- Heavy cream, .5 c

- Chicken stock, .5 c

- Minced garlic, 2 tsp.

- Butter, 2 tbsp.

- Pepper

- Salt

- Skin on, bone-in chicken thighs, 4

What to Do

1. You need to warm your oven to 400.

2. Put a skillet that can go into the oven on top of the stove on medium heat. Add in one tablespoon of butter. Sprinkle the chicken with pepper and salt.

3. Lay the chicken in the skillet and brown on both sides. This will take about six minutes.

4. Take thighs out of skillet and place to the side on a plate.

5. Add the rest of the butter and add garlic until fragrant and translucent.

6. Add lemon juice, heavy cream, and chicken stock. Mix well. Allow to boil and put the chicken back into the skillet.

7. Cover and place into the oven for 30 minutes.

Stuffed Chicken Breast

This recipe makes 4 servings and contains 389 calories; 30 grams fat; 25 grams protein; 3 grams net carbohydrates per serving

What You Need

- EVOO, 2 tbsp.

- Boneless, skin on chicken breasts, 4

- Chopped basil, 2 tbsp.

- Roasted, chopped bell pepper, .25 c

- Chopped Kalamata olives, .25 c

- Room temperature goat cheese, .5 c

- Chopped onion, .25 c

- Butter, 1 tbsp.

What to Do

1. You need to warm your oven to 400.

2. Place a skillet on top of the stove and melt butter on medium heat.

3. Mix in the onion, cooking until translucent.

4. Put the basil, bell pepper, olives, cheese, and onion into a blow. Mix well to combine. Place in the refrigerator for 30 minutes.

5. Cut pockets into each of the chicken breasts, place the filling inside each breast. Secure with toothpicks.

6. Using the same skillet, warm up the olive oil. Sear the chicken on each side.

7. Place into the oven for 15 minutes. Chicken is done when it reaches an internal temperature of 165.

8. Carefully remove toothpicks and enjoy.

Turkey Rissoles

This recipe makes 4 servings and contains 440 calories; 34 grams fat; 27 grams protein; 3 grams net carbohydrates per serving

What You Need

- Olive oil, 2 tbsp.

- Ground almonds, 1 c

- Pepper

- Salt

- Minced garlic, 1 tsp.

- Chopped scallion, 1

- Ground turkey, 1 lb.

What to Do

1. You need to warm your oven to 350.

2. Place the pepper, salt, garlic, scallion, and turkey into a bowl. With your hands, mix everything together.

3. Shape into eight patties and flatten.

4. Place the almonds in a shallow bowl and put the patties into the almonds to coat. Press gently to make sure the almonds stick to the patties.

5. Put a skillet onto the stove and warm the olive oil on medium heat. Place the patties into the skillet and cook for ten minutes on each side.

6. Place aluminum foil onto a baking sheet. Lay the patties on a cooking sheet and slide into the oven. Bake for eight minutes. Turn oven and cook for an additional eight minutes.

Stuffed Pork Chops

This recipe makes 4 servings and contains 481 calories; 38 grams fat; 29 grams protein; 2 grams net carbohydrates per serving

What You Need

- Olive oil, 2 tbsp.

- Pepper

- Salt

- Butterflied pork chops, 4

- Chopped thyme, 1 tsp.

- Chopped almonds, .25 c

- Chopped walnuts, .5 c

- Goat cheese, 3 oz.

What to Do

1. You need to warm your oven to 400.

2. Put the thyme, almonds, walnuts, goat cheese into a bowl. Stir well to combine.

3. Sprinkle pepper and salt on the pork chops on all sides. Spread the stuffing on one side of the pork chop. Fold the other side over and secure with toothpicks.

4. Place a large skillet on top of the stove and warm the olive oil on medium heat. Sear the pork chops until browned on each side. This will take about ten minutes.

5. Lay this in a baking dish and cook for 20 minutes.

6. Carefully remove the toothpicks and enjoy.

Rosemary Garlic Rack of Lamb

This recipe makes 4 servings and contains 354 calories; 30 grams fat; 21 grams protein; 0 gram net carbohydrates per serving

What You Need

- French-cut rack of lamb, 1 lb.

- Salt

- Minced garlic, 2 tsp.

- Chopped rosemary, 2 tbsp.

- EVOO, 4 tbsp.

What to Do

1. Add the salt, garlic, rosemary, and olive oil into a bowl. Mix well to combine.

2. Put the lamb into a zip-top bag and pour in the olive oil mixture. Rub the lamb with the mixture until coated. Press out as much air as you can get and make sure it is sealed.

3. Refrigerate for at least two hours.

4. To cook, take out of the refrigerator and let it cool to room temperature for 20 minutes.

5. You need to warm your oven to 450.

6. Put a skillet that can go into the oven on top of the stove and let it get hot. Sear the rack of lamb on each side. This will take about five minutes.

7. Sit the rack upright in the skillet and interlace the bones. Place into the oven for about 20 minutes. This will get them to a medium rare consistency. The internal temp will be around 125.

8. Allow to sit for ten minutes and cut into chops.

9. Each person gets four chops.

Garlic Short Ribs

This recipe makes 4 servings and contains 481 calories; 38 grams fat; 29 grams protein; 2 grams net carbohydrates per serving

What You Need

- Beef broth, 3 c

- Dry red wine, .5 c

- Minced garlic, 2 tsp.

- Olive oil, 1 tbsp.

- Pepper

- Salt

- Beef short ribs, 4 – 4 oz.

What to Do

1. You need to warm your oven to 325.

2. Sprinkle pepper and salt on the ribs on all sides.

3. Put a large skillet that can go into the oven on top of the stove on medium heat and warm up the olive oil.

4. Sear the ribs on every side and place on a plate.

5. Using the same skillet, put the garlic in and cook until softened around three minutes.

6. Add in the red wine and whisk to deglaze. Simmer until wine is reduced slightly.

7. Add in ribs, juices on plate, and beef broth. And allow it to boil.

8. Cover and put the skillet into the oven for two hours.

9. Remove ribs onto a serving platter and drizzle with cooking liquid.

Bacon Wrapped Steaks

This recipe makes 4 servings and contains 565 calories; 49 grams fat; 28 grams protein; 0 gram net carbohydrates per serving

What You Need

- Pepper

- Salt

- EVOO, 1 tbsp.

- Sliced bacon, 8

- Beef steaks, 4 – 4 oz.

What to Do

1. You need to warm your oven to 450.

2. Sprinkle each steak with pepper and salt generously.

3. Wrap two slices of bacon around the edge of each steak. Secure with toothpicks.

4. Place a large skillet on top of the stove and warm the olive oil.

5. Sear the steaks on each side for four minutes. Place them on a cooking sheet.

6. Bake them in the oven for six minutes for medium doneness.

7. Take out of the oven and allow to rest for ten minutes.

8. Carefully remove toothpicks and enjoy.

Italian Burgers

This recipe makes 4 servings and contains 441 calories; 37 grams fat; 22 grams protein; 3 grams net carbohydrates per serving

What You Need

- Thinly sliced small onion

- Minced garlic, 1 tsp.

- Thickly sliced tomato

- Olive oil, 1 tbsp.

- Salt, .25 tsp.

- Chopped basil, 2 tbsp.

- Ground almonds, .25 c

- Ground beef, 1 lb.

What to Do

1. Place the salt, garlic, basil, ground almonds, and ground beef into a bowl. Use your hand to combine all ingredients.

2. Divide into four equal portions and form into patties. Flatten to about one-half inch thickness.

3. Put a large cast iron skillet on top of the stove and warm the olive oil on medium heat.

4. Place the burgers into the skillet and cook for six minutes on each side.

5. Place onto paper towels to drain. Whisk away any grease that might form on the top of each burger with paper towels.

6. Serve with onion and tomato.

Saffron Shrimp

This recipe makes 2 servings and contains 333 calories; 13 grams fat; 45 grams protein; 9 grams net carbohydrates per serving

What You Need

- Lemon juice, 1 tbsp.

- Cayenne

- White pepper

- Chicken broth, .5 c

- Chopped tomato, 1

- Paprika

- Saffron

- Minced garlic, 2 cloves

- Cooked shrimp, 1 lb.

- Chopped fennel, .5

- Ghee, 2 tbsp.

What to Do

1. Place a large skillet on top of the stove and melt the ghee on medium heat. Put the fennel into the skillet and cook until soft. Add in the paprika, saffron, garlic, and shrimp. Cook until shrimp is turning pink. If the skillet gets dry, add more ghee.

2. Add in pepper, cayenne, lemon juice, broth, and tomato. Bring to simmer and let the liquid reduce for 20 minutes. Enjoy.

Pesto Chicken Casserole

This recipe makes 4 servings and contains 512 calories; 110 grams fat; 42 grams protein; 7 grams net carbohydrates per serving

What You Need

- Pepper

- Salt

- Diced feta, 8 oz.

- Chopped garlic, 1 clove

- Chopped olives, .5 c

- Heavy whipping cream, 1.5 c

- Olive oil, 4 tbsp.

- Leafy greens, .75 c

- Chicken breasts, 1.5 lbs.

- Pesto, .33 c

- Butter, 4 tbsp.

What to Do

1. You need to warm your oven to 450.

2. Chop the chicken into cubes and sprinkle with pepper and salt.

3. Place a skillet on top of the stove on medium heat and melt butter. Cook the chicken until browned. Do this in batches until all have been browned.

4. Add the pesto and cream to a bowl and mix well to combine.

5. Place the cooked chicken to the bottom of a casserole dish. Add in the olives, feta, and garlic. Drizzle the pesto over everything.

6. Slide into the oven and cook for 25 minutes until the edges are browned and bubbly.

Meat Pie

This recipe makes 6 servings and contains 133 calories; 47 grams fat; 38 grams protein; 7 grams net carbohydrates per serving

What You Need

- Chopped onion, .5

- Minced garlic, 1 clove

- Butter, 2 tbsp.

- Ground beef, 1.5 lb.

- Pepper

- Salt

- Water, .5 c

- Dried oregano, 1 tbsp.

- Tomato paste, 4 tbsp.

- For the Crust:

- Almond flour, .75 c

- Water, 4 tbsp.

- Sesame seeds, 4 tbsp.

- Egg, 1

- Coconut flour, 4 tbsp.

- Salt

- Ground psyllium husk powder, 1 tbsp.

- Baking powder, 1 tsp.

- For the Topping:

- Shredded cheese, 7 oz.

- Cottage cheese, 8 oz.

What to Do

1. You need to warm your oven to 350.

2. Place a skillet on top of the stove on medium and warm the butter. Mix in the garlic and onion, cooking until soft.

3. Mix in the beef, cooking until completely browned. Add in the salt, basil, pepper, and oregano. Stir together.

4. Pour in the water and tomato paste. Mix well. Lower heat and simmer 20 minutes. While cooking, make the crust.

5. Add the dough ingredients to a food processor and mix until it forms a ball. You can do this by hand if you don't have a food processor.

6. Take a springform pan and grease it generously. Place a piece of parchment paper into the bottom.

7. Spread the dough onto the bottom and sides with your greased fingers.

8. Place into the oven and bake for 15 minutes. Pour meat mixture into the crust.

9. Mix the topping ingredients and spread on top the of meat. Let the pie bake for 35 minutes until golden.

Soups

Cauliflower Soup

This recipe makes 8 servings and contains 227 calories; 21 grams fat; 8 grams protein; 2 grams net carbohydrates per serving

What You Need

- Butter, .25 c

- Shredded cheddar, 1 c

- Pepper

- Salt

- Heavy cream, 1 c

- Nutmeg, .5 tsp.

- Chicken stock, 4 c

- Chopped cauliflower, 1 head

- Chopped onion, .5

What to Do

1. Add the butter to a pot and melt.

2. Cook the cauliflower and onion together for about ten minutes.

3. Mix in the nutmeg and chicken stock and allow everything to come to a boil. Lower to a simmer and cook for 15 minutes.

4. Mix in the heavy cream.

5. Add the soup to a blender and puree until smooth. You may need to do this in more than one batch. Alternatively, you can use an immersion blender if you have one.

6. Pour the soup back into the pot and season with some pepper and salt. Top with the cheese and serve.

Thai Chicken Soup

This recipe makes 4 servings and contains 324 calories; 19 grams fat; 23 grams protein; 13 grams net carbohydrates per serving

What You Need

- Bunch cilantro

- Thai chili paste, 1 tsp.

- Lime juice, 2 tbsp.

- Cubed tomatoes, 2

- Sliced mushrooms, 1 c

- Thai fish sauce, 1 tbsp.

- Kaffir lime leaves, 6

- White parts from fresh lemongrass, 2 stalks – chopped and crushed

- Galangal, thumb-sized chunk

- Diced chicken thighs, 1 lb.

- Chicken broth, 14 oz.

- Coconut milk, 14 oz.

What to Do

1. Add the lemongrass, sliced galangal, chili paste, broth, and coconut milk to a pot and heat to medium-high. Allow this to come to a boil.

2. Mix in the chicken and cook for another two minutes. Lower the heat.

3. Mix in the tomatoes and mushrooms. Cook for another three to five minutes.

4. Mix in the lime juice and fish sauce.

5. Break up the lime leaves and stir them into the soup.

6. Remove the galangal and lemongrass. Serve the soup topped with some fresh cilantro.

Bacon Cheeseburger Soup

This recipe makes 4 servings and contains 758 calories; 57 grams fat; 48 grams protein; 11 grams net carbohydrates per serving

What You Need

- Pepper, .5 tsp.

- Salt, 2 tsp.

- Chili powder, 1 tsp.

- Onion powder, .5 tsp.

- Cream cheese, 3 oz.

- Dried parsley, 1 tsp.

- Heavy cream, .5 c

- Shredded cheddar, 1 c

- Beef broth, 4 c

- Butter, 3 tbsp.

- Garlic powder, .5 tsp.

- Bacon, 4 slices

- Ground beef, 1 lb.

What to Do

1. Add the bacon to a large pot and cook until crispy. Lay it out on paper towels to drain.

2. Add in the spices, beef, and butter. Let this cook until the beef has browned. Make sure you break it apart as it cooks.

3. Add in the cheddar cheese, cream cheese, tomato paste, and broth. Stir until everything is melted and combined.

4. Cook the soup, covered, on low for 25 minutes

5. Sprinkle in some pepper and salt. Garnish the soup with the crumbled cooked bacon and some heavy cream.

Cheesy Broccoli Soup

This recipe makes 4 servings and contains 185 calories; 14 grams fat; 10 grams protein; 4 grams net carbohydrates per serving

What You Need

- Pepper
- Salt
- Shredded cheddar, 1 c
- Broccoli, 3 c
- Heavy cream, .25 c
- Cream cheese, 1 tbsp.
- Chicken broth, 4 c
- Minced garlic, 2 cloves
- Diced small onion

What to Do

1. Melt the butter in a pot and sauté the onions for three to four minutes. Mix in the garlic, cooking until fragrant.
2. Mix in the broccoli and chicken broth.
3. Allow the mixture to come to a boil and then reduce the heat so that it simmers for a few minutes.
4. After the broccoli is soft, puree the soup with an immersion blender.
5. Mix in the cream cheese and cream, stirring until well combined and melted.
6. Take the pot off the heat and mix in the cheddar cheese. Enjoy.

Beef Stew

This recipe makes 4 servings and contains 706 calories; 57 grams fat; 37 grams protein; 6 grams net carbohydrates per serving

What You Need

- Pepper

- Salt

- Almond flour, .25 c

- Thyme, 1 tbsp.

- Worcestershire sauce, 1 tbsp.

- Beef broth, 1 c

- Diced tomatoes, 3

- Minced garlic, 2 cloves

- Hot sauce, 2 tsp.

- Chopped onion, .5

- 1-inch cube beef stew meat, 2 lbs.

What to Do

1. Turn your slow cooker to the high settings.

2. Mix the almond flour with some pepper and salt. Coat the stew meat in the flour. Lay the meat in your slow cooker.

3. Pour in the remaining ingredients.

4. Set to cook for 30 minutes on high, then switch to low and cook for six hours.

5. Adjust the flavorings as you see fit.

Chicken Soup

This recipe makes 8 servings and contains 285 calories; 40 grams fat; 33 grams protein; 4 grams net carbohydrates per serving

What You Need

- Butter, .5 c

- Celery stalks, 2

- Dried parsley, 2 tsp.

- Sliced mushrooms, 6 oz.

- Minced garlic, 2 cloves

- Dried onion, 2 tbsp.

- Salt, 1 tsp.

- Chicken broth, 8 c

- Sliced cabbage, 2 c

- Pepper, .25 tsp.

- Shredded, cooked chicken, 2 c

- Medium Carrot

What to Do

1. Place a large stock pot to the stove on medium and melt butter. Slice the celery and carrots.

2. Put the dried onion, mushrooms, celery, and garlic into the pot and cook for four minutes.

3. Add in salt, parsley, pepper, chicken, broth, and carrot. Allow this to boil for 12 minutes or until cabbage is tender.

Easy Chicken Chili

This recipe makes 4 servings and contains 421 calories; 21 grams fat; 45 grams protein; 6 grams net carbohydrates per serving

What You Need

- Pepper

- Salt

- Cream cheese, 4 oz.

- Chili powder, 1 tbsp.

- Serrano pepper, 1

- Garlic powder, .5 tbsp.

- Cumin, 1 tbsp.

- Tomato puree, 2 oz.

- Diced tomatoes, 8 oz.

- Chicken broth, 2 c

- Onion, .5

- Butter, 1 tbsp.

- Boneless, skinless, chicken breasts, 4

What to Do

1. Take the chicken breasts and cut them into cubes.

2. Place a large pan on medium heat. Pour water into a pan and allow to boil. Add chicken into the water and boil until cooked through about ten minutes. Remove chicken from pan and set to the side. Pour water out of the pan and place back onto heat.

3. Add butter to melt. Add onion and cook until softened. Put chicken back into the pot along with the chili powder, broth, tomato puttee, garlic,

Serrano pepper, cumin, and tomatoes. Let everything boil. Turn to a simmer for ten minutes.

4. While chili is simmering, cut the cream cheese into chunks and place in the pan. Stirring until melted.

5. Ladle into bowls and enjoy.

Turkey and Leek Soup

This recipe makes 4 servings and contains 305 calories; 11 grams fat; 15 grams protein; 3 grams net carbohydrates per serving

What You Need

- Shredded turkey, 3 c

- Chopped zoodles, 3 c

- Chopped parsley, .25 c

- Pepper

- Salt

- Chicken broth, 6 c

- Butter, 1 tbsp.

- Chopped leeks, 2

- Chopped celery, 3

What to Do

1. Place a large stock pot on medium and melt butter. Add in celery and leeks, cooking until softened for about five minutes.

2. Add in chicken broth, pepper, salt, turkey meat, and parsley into the pot. Once this comes to a boil, turn to a simmer for 20 minutes.

3. Add in the zoodles and cook an additional five minutes.

4. Ladle into bowls and enjoy.

Turkey Chili

This recipe makes 5 servings and contains 295 calories; 15 grams fat; 25 grams protein; 4 grams net carbohydrates per serving

What You Need

- Chili powder, 2 tbsp.

- Pepper

- Salt

- Cumin, 1 tbsp.

- Turmeric, 1 tbsp.

- Grated ginger, 2 tbsp.

- Coconut oil, 2 tbsp.

- Coriander, 1 tbsp.

- Sliced onions, 2

- Minced garlic, 2 cloves

- Coconut cream, 2 tbsp.

- Diced tomatoes, 20 oz.

- Kale, 3 oz.

- Cooked and shredded turkey breasts, 18 oz.

What to Do

1. Place a large pot on medium and melt coconut oil. Add the onion, cooking until soft. Mix in ginger and garlic and cook until fragrant about one minute.

2. Put the chili powder, cumin, salt, coriander, turmeric, pepper, and tomatoes into the pot and stir well to combine. Add in the coconut cream. Bring to boil and cook for ten minutes.

3. Add in the kale and turkey breasts. Allow this to boil and then simmer for another 15 minutes.

Turkey Stew

This recipe makes 6 servings and contains 193 calories; 11 grams fat; 27 grams protein; 2 grams net carbohydrates per serving

What You Need

- Chopped cilantro, 1 tbsp.

- Sour cream, .25 c

- Cumin, 2 tsp.

- Coriander, 1 tsp.

- Salsa verde, .5 c

- Garlic powder, .5 tsp.

- Chopped canned chipotle peppers, 1 tbsp.

- Pepper

- Salt

- Chicken broth, 6 c

- Green beans, 2 c

- Shredded, cooked turkey meat, 4 c

What to Do

1. Add the broth to a pot.

2. Add the green beans, cooking for ten minutes.

3. Mix in the pepper, cumin, chipotles, salsa verde, salt, coriander, garlic powder, and turkey. Stir well and cook another ten minutes.

4. Add in sour cream and give everything a good stir. Take off heat and divide into bowls. Sprinkle with cilantro and serve.

Coconut Chicken Soup

This recipe makes 4 servings and contains 387 calories; 23 grams fat; 31 grams protein; 5 grams net carbohydrates per serving

What You Need

- Chopped celery, .25 c

- Coconut cream, .5 c

- Pepper

- Salt

- Chicken broth, 4 c

- Diced chicken breasts, 2

- Cream cheese, 4 oz.

- Butter, 3 tbsp.

What to Do

1. Melt the butter in a large pot. Add in celery, cooking until soft. Mix in the pepper, salt, cream cheese, and coconut cream. Stir until cream cheese is melted and everything is well incorporated.

2. Stir in chicken and simmer for 15 minutes.

3. Ladle into bowls and serve.

Mexican Turkey Soup

This recipe makes 4 servings and contains 387 calories; 24 grams fat; 38 grams protein; 6 grams net carbohydrates per serving

What You Need

- Chunked cheddar, 8 oz.

- Chunky salsa, 15 oz.

- Chicken broth, 15 oz.

- Cubed turkey thighs, 1.5 lbs.

What to Do

1. Put everything in a slow cooker and mix.

2. Cover, turn to high and cook for four hours. You can also cook this on low for eight hours.

3. Gently remove the lid, stir well to incorporate the cheese.

4. Ladle into bowls and serve.

Sun-Dried Tomato and Chicken Stew

This recipe makes 4 servings and contains 224 calories; 11 grams fat; 23 grams protein; 6 grams net carbohydrates per serving

What You Need

- Pepper

- Salt

- Heavy cream, .5 c

- Thyme, .25 tsp.

- Oregano, .5 tsp.

- Spinach, 1 c

- Chopped sun-dried tomatoes, 2 oz.

- Rosemary, .5 tsp.

- Minced garlic, 3 cloves

- Cubed chicken thighs, 28 oz.

- Chopped shallot, 1

- Chicken broth, 2 c

- Chopped celery, 2

- Chopped carrots, 2

- Xanthan gum, pinch

What to Do

1. Heat a large pot and add in the pepper, oregano, garlic, celery, onion, thyme, salt, rosemary, carrots, tomatoes, broth, and chicken. Stir well to combine.

2. Let this come to a boil and then turn to a simmer for 45 minutes.

3. Do a taste test and adjust pepper and salt if needed. Add in the spinach, xanthan gum, and cream. Cook an additional ten minutes.

4. Ladle into bowls and serve.

Cream of Tomato and Thyme Soup

This recipe makes 6 servings and contains 310 calories; 27 grams fat; 11 grams protein; 3 grams net carbohydrates per serving

What You Need

- Heavy cream, 1 c

- Pepper

- Salt

- Water, 1.5 c

- Thyme leaves, 1 tsp.

- Canned tomatoes, 2 – 28 oz.

- Diced cashews, .5 c

- Diced onion, 2 large

- Ghee, 2 tbsp.

What to Do

1. Melt the ghee in a large pot. Add in the onion and cook until soft.

2. Add in pepper, salt, cashews, water, thyme, and tomatoes. Stir to combine. Bring to boil. Cover with a lid and simmer it for ten minutes.

3. Take the lid off. Use an immersion blender to process until smooth. Taste and adjust if necessary. Add in the heavy cream, stir well to combine.

4. Ladle into bowls and serve.

Gazpacho

This recipe makes 6 servings and contains 528 calories; 46 grams fat; 8 grams protein; 8 grams net carbohydrates per serving

What You Need

- Salt

- Apple cider vinegar, 2 tbsp.

- Chopped onion, 1 small

- Goat cheese, 7 oz.

- Chopped tomatoes, 4

- Roasted green bell peppers, 2

- Lemon juice, 2 tbsp.

- Olive oil, 1 c

- Chopped cucumber, 1

- Chopped green onion, 2

- Garlic, 2 cloves

- Avocados, 2

- Roasted red bell peppers, 2

What to Do

1. Place the salt, vinegar, olive oil, lemon juice, garlic, onion, avocado, tomatoes, and peppers into a blender or food processor. Process until either completely smooth or slightly chunky. Whichever you would prefer.

2. Taste and adjust seasonings as needed.

3. Place into an airtight container. Add in the green onions and cucumbers. Refrigerate for no less than two hours.

4. When ready to eat, ladle into bowls.

5. Top with a drizzle of olive oil and goat cheese.

Coconut and Shrimp Curry Soup

This recipe makes 4 servings and contains 375 calories; 35 grams fat; 9 grams protein; 2 grams net carbohydrates per serving

What You Need

- Halved green beans, 1 bunch

- Chili pepper

- Salt

- Coconut milk, 6 oz.

- Red curry paste, 2 tbsp.

- Ginger garlic pureed, 2 tsp.

- Peeled and deveined jumbo shrimp, 1 lb.

- Ghee, 2 tbsp.

What to Do

1. Place a skillet on medium and melt ghee. Add in the shrimp and sprinkle with pepper and salt. Cool until turning slightly pink. Take out of the skillet and put on a plate. Set to the side.

2. Add the red curry paste and ginger garlic puree to the same skillet and cook until fragrant.

3. Add in the green beans, chili pepper, salt, coconut milk, and place the shrimp back into the skillet. Stir well to combine. Cook an additional four minutes. Lower heat and simmer another three minutes, stir occasionally.

4. Adjust any of the seasonings that you need to.

5. Ladle into bowls and serve with some cauli-rice if desired.

Green Minestrone Soup

This recipe makes 4 servings and contains 227 calories; 20 grams fat; 8 grams protein; 2 grams net carbohydrates per serving

What You Need

- Pepper

- Salt

- Baby spinach, 1 c

- Vegetable broth, 5 c

- Chopped celery, 2

- Chopped broccoli, 2 heads

- Onion garlic puree, 2 tbsp.

- Ghee, 2 tbsp.

What to Do

1. Place a saucepan on medium and melt ghee. Add in the onion-garlic puree and cook until warmed.

2. Mix in the celery and broccoli and cook until tender.

3. Pour in broth and stir everything together. Let this come up to a boil. Lower the heat and cook while covered for five minutes.

4. Add spinach in batches until wilted. Add pepper and salt to taste and cook four more minutes. Taste and adjust seasoning if needed.

5. Ladle into bowls and sprinkle with Gruyere cheese if desired. Can be eaten with a low carb bread.

Shrimp Stew

This recipe makes 6 servings and contains 324 calories; 21 grams fat; 23 grams protein; 5 grams net carbohydrates per serving

What You Need

- Pepper

- Salt

- Chopped Dill

- Chopped cilantro, .25 c

- Chopped onions, .25 c

- Sriracha sauce, 2 tbsp.

- Diced tomatoes, 14 oz.

- Minced garlic, 1 clove

- Olive oil, .25 c

- Peeled, deveined shrimp, 1.5 lb.

- Diced roasted peppers, .25 c

- Lime juice, 2 tbsp.

- Coconut milk, 1 c

What to Do

1. Place a pot on medium and warm olive oil. Mix in the onion, cooking until translucent.

2. Mix in garlic, cooking until fragrant.

3. Add in cilantro, shrimp, and tomatoes. Cook until shrimp turns pink.

4. Stir in coconut milk and Sriracha and cook a few more minutes. Don't boil, just warm through. Add in lime juice and sprinkle with pepper and salt. Taste and adjust any seasonings as needed.

5. Ladle into bowls, sprinkle with fresh dill and serve.

Sausage Beer Soup

This recipe makes 8 servings and contains 244 calories; 17 grams fat; 5 grams protein; 4 grams net carbohydrates per serving

What You Need

- Chopped cilantro

- Pepper

- Salt

- Cheddar cheese, 1 c

- Diced onion, 1

- Chopped celery, 1 c

- Beef broth, 2 c

- Beer, 6 oz.

- Red pepper flakes, 1 tsp.

- Cream cheese, 8 oz.

- Minced garlic, 4 cloves

- Chopped carrots, 1 c

- Sliced beef sausages, 10 oz.

- Heavy cream, 1 c

What to Do

1. Turn your slow cooker to low.

2. Add the pepper, salt, red pepper flakes, salt, celery, onion, carrots, sausage, beer, and broth into the slow cooker. Stir well to combine. Add in just enough water to cover the ingredients by two inches.

3. Put the lid on the cooker and set the timer for six hours.

4. Carefully remove the lid and add in the cream cheese, cheddar, and heavy cream. Stir well. Place the lid back on and cook an additional two hours.

5. When done, stir well to combine. Taste and adjust seasonings if needed.

6. Ladle into bowls, sprinkle with cilantro and serve.

Wild Mushroom and Thyme Soup

This recipe makes 4 servings and contains 281 calories; 25 grams fat; 6 grams protein; 6 grams net carbohydrates per serving

What You Need

- Pepper

- Salt

- Chicken broth, 4 c

- Minced garlic, 2 cloves

- Thyme leaves, 2 tsp.

- Chopped wild mushrooms, 12 oz.

- Crème Fraiche, 5 oz.

- Butter, .25 c

What to Do

1. Melt the ghee in a large pot. Add in the garlic and cook until fragrant. Put the mushrooms into the pot and sprinkle with pepper and salt. Cook for ten minutes. Add in broth and allow to boil.

2. Lower heat and simmer for ten minutes. Use an immersion blender and process until smooth. You can also use a blender if you don't have an immersion blender.

3. Put the crème Fraiche in and stir well.

4. Ladle into bowls and garnish with thyme.

Reuben Soup

This recipe makes 7 servings and contains 450 calories; 37 grams fat; 23 grams protein; 8 grams net carbohydrates per serving

What You Need

- Pepper

- Salt

- Swiss cheese, 1.5 c

- Butter, 3 tbsp.

- Chopped corned beef, 1 lb.

- Sauerkraut, 1 c

- Heavy cream, 2 c

- Minced garlic, 2 cloves

- Diced celery, 2

- Caraway seeds, 1 tsp.

- Diced onion, 1

What to Do

1. Place a large pot on medium and melt butter. Mix in the onion and celery, cooking until tender. Mix in the garlic and cook until fragrant.

2. Add in broth, pepper, caraway seeds, salt, and sauerkraut. Stir well. Allow to boil. Lower heat and put corned beef into the pot.

3. Simmer for 15 minutes. Taste and adjust seasonings if needed.

4. Add in cheese and heavy cream and cook one more minute.

Salads

Taco Salad

This recipe makes 4 servings and contains 516 calories; 37 grams fat; 35 grams protein; 5 grams net carbohydrates per serving

What You Need

- Water, .5 c

- Cumin, 1.5 tsp.

- Paprika, .5 tsp.

- Oregano, .25 tsp.

- Garlic powder, .25 tsp.

- Ground beef, 1 lb.

- Sliced onion, 2 tbsp.

- Salt, 1 tsp.

- Sour cream, .5 c

- Olive oil, 1 tbsp.

- Juice of lime, .5

- Avocado

- Chopped tomato

- Chopped lettuce, 2 c

- Grated cheese, .5 c

What to Do

1. Add the beef to a skillet and brown. This will take about eight to ten minutes.

2. Mix in the cumin, paprika, oregano, garlic powder, and ½ cup of water. Allow this to simmer for three minutes, or until the water has evaporated.

3. Toss together the onion, avocado, and lettuce.

4. Mix in the salt, lime juice, and oil.

5. Top with the beef, cheese, tomatoes, and sour cream.

Crab Salad Avocado

This recipe makes 2 servings and contains 389 calories; 31 grams fat; 19 grams protein; 5 grams net carbohydrates per serving

What You Need

- Pepper
- Salt .
- Chopped cilantro, 1 tsp.
- Chopped scallion, .5
- Chopped English cucumber, .25 c
- Chopped red bell pepper, .25 c
- Cream cheese, .5 c
- Crab meat, 4.5 oz.
- Lemon juice, .5 tsp.
- Halved avocado

What to Do

1. Brush the avocado with the lemon so that it doesn't become brown. Lay them on a plate cut side up.
2. Mix together the pepper, salt, cilantro, scallion, cucumber, red pepper, crab meat, and cream cheese.
3. Divide the crabmeat mixture between the two avocado halves and serve.

Tuna Salad

This recipe makes 2 servings and contains 465 calories; 18 grams fat; 68 grams protein; 6 grams net carbohydrates per serving

What You Need

- Salt, 1 tsp.

- Mayonnaise, 2 tbsp.

- EVOO, 1 tbsp.

- Lemon juice, 2 tbsp.

- Chopped cilantro, .5 bunch

- Sliced small onion

- Dijon, 2 tsp.

- Sliced cucumber, .5

- Chopped boiled eggs, 2

- Drained tuna in oil, 2 15-oz. can

What to Do

1. Mix together the salt, olive oil, lemon juice, Dijon, and mayonnaise.

2. Toss everything together. Top with the dressing and toss everything together. Enjoy.

BLT Salad

This recipe makes 4 servings and contains 228 calories; 18 grams fat; 1 gram protein; 2 grams net carbohydrates per serving

What You Need

- Sliced cooked chicken breast
- Toasted sesame seeds, 1 tsp.
- Chopped hardboiled egg, 2
- Chopped cooked bacon, 6 slices
- Chopped tomato
- Sunflower seeds, 1 tbsp.
- Shredded lettuce, 4 c
- Pepper
- Red wine vinegar, 2 tbsp.
- Bacon fat, 2 tbsp.

What to Do

1. Whisk the vinegar and bacon fat together until emulsified. Add in the pepper.
2. Toss the tomato and lettuce into the dressing.
3. Divide this between four plates and top each with chicken, sesame seeds, sunflower seeds, egg, and bacon.

Salmon Salad

This recipe makes 2 servings and contains 492 calories; 39 grams fat; 25 grams protein; 7 grams net carbohydrates per serving

What You Need

- Pepper, .5 tsp.

- Salt, .25 tsp.

- Olive oil, 2 tbsp.

- Chopped walnuts, .25 c

- Diced avocado

- Smoked salmon, 7 oz.

- Lemon juice, 2 tbsp.

- Mixed leafy greens, 6 oz.

What to Do

1. Add the pepper, salt, avocado, and leafy greens to a bowl and toss everything together.

2. Add in the lemon juice and olive oil and mix everything together.

3. Divide into two serving bowls and top with the walnuts and salmon.

Feta Salad

This recipe makes 2 servings and contains 619 calories; 59 grams fat; 13 grams protein; 8 grams net carbohydrates per serving

What You Need

- Salt, .5 tsp.

- EVOO, .25 c

- Pepper, .25 tsp.

- Dijon, 1 tsp.

- Balsamic vinegar, 2 tbsp.

- Bacon, 2 slices

- Feta, 3 oz.

- Walnut pieces, .5 c

- Mixed salad greens, 2 c

What to Do

1. Cook the bacon until crispy.

2. Mix the walnuts, cheese, and greens together. Crumble up the bacon and toss into the greens.

3. Beat together the pepper, salt, mustard, and balsamic vinegar. Whisk the dressing as you pour in the olive oil until well blended.

4. Dress the salad and toss everything together. Serve.

Turkey and Avocado Salad

This recipe makes 4 servings and contains 559 calories; 30 grams fat; 60 grams protein; 5 grams net carbohydrates per serving

What You Need

- Pepper

- Salt

- Sliced cherry tomatoes, 12

- Mustard, 1 tbsp.

- Olive oil, 2 tbsp.

- Spinach, 7 c

- Cubed avocado, 1 c

- Crumbled feta, 1 c

- Chopped cooked turkey bacon, 3 slices

- Diced grilled turkey breasts, 2 lb.

What to Do

1. Mix together the oil, mustard, and a tablespoon of water. Stir in some pepper and salt. Set to the side.

2. Toss the spinach in half of the dressing.

3. Add in the tomatoes, cheese, avocado, turkey, and bacon.

4. Add in the rest of the dressing and sprinkle in some pepper and salt. Enjoy.

Caesar Salad

This recipe makes 2 servings and contains 734 calories; 58 grams fat; 41 grams protein; 6 grams net carbohydrates per serving

What You Need

- Homemade Caesar dressing, 2 tbsp.

- Parmesan, 1 tbsp.

- Romaine lettuce, 4 c

- Bacon, 1 c

- Sliced avocado

- Grilled chicken breast, 10 oz.

For the Dressing

- Lemon juice, 2 tbsp.

- Garlic clove

- Pepper

- Salt

- Mayonnaise, .5 c

- Dijon, 1.5 tsp.

What to Do

1. To make the salad dressing, add everything to a blender and combine until smooth.

2. To make the salad, cook the chopped bacon and heat until crispy.

3. Mix together the cooked bacon, chicken, and sliced avocado.

4. Drizzle the salad with the Caesar dressing. Top with some Parmesan and enjoy.

Brussels Sprouts Salad

This recipe makes 1 serving, and contains 282 calories; 28 grams fat; 3 grams protein; 5 grams net carbohydrates per serving

What You Need

- Pepper

- Lemon juice, 1 tbsp.

- EVOO, 2 tbsp.

- Chopped Brussels, 1 c

What to Do

1. Place the lemon juice, olive oil, and Brussels into a bowl. Toss to coat. Sprinkle on some pepper, taste and adjust seasoning if needed.

Avocado Salad

This recipe makes 4 servings and contains 285 calories; 123 grams fat; 27 grams protein; 6 grams net carbohydrates per serving

What You Need

- Goat cheese, 8 oz.

- Sliced bacon, 8 oz.

- Avocados, 2

- Arugula, .5 c

- Walnuts, 4 oz.

- For Dressing:

- Juice of .5 lemon

- Heavy whipping cream, 2 tbsp.

- Mayonnaise, .5 c

- Olive oil, .5 c

What to Do

1. You need to warm your oven to 400. Use parchment paper to line a baking dish.

2. Slice the goat cheese into slices that are one half inches thick and lay in the baking dish.

3. Place into the oven and bake until golden.

4. Place a skillet on top of the stove and cook the bacon until crispy.

5. Slice the avocados in half and carefully remove the pit. Scoop out and slice.

6. Divide the arugula evenly between four plates. Add the sliced avocado on top. Place the bacon and goat cheese on top. Sprinkle with walnuts.

7. Add the dressing ingredients to a blender and mix until smooth. Add in some pepper and salt. Serve with a drizzle of dressing.

Tuna Salad

This recipe makes 2 servings and contains 387 calories; 91 grams fat; 33 grams protein; 6 grams net carbohydrates per serving

What You Need

- Pepper

- Salt

- Romaine lettuce, .5 lb.

- Dijon mustard, 1 tsp.

- Cherry tomatoes, 4 oz.

- Eggs, 4

- Juice and zest from .5 lemon

- Scallions, 2

- Olive oil, 2 tbsp.

- Mayonnaise, .75 c

- Celery stalks, 4 oz.

- Tuna, 5 oz.

What to Do

1. Finely chop the celery and scallions. Combine the lemon zest, lemon juice, mayonnaise, mustard, celery, scallions, and tuna. Add pepper and salt. Set to the side.

2. Put the eggs into a pot and cover with water. Let the eggs boil for six minutes for soft or medium eggs or ten minutes for hardboiled.

3. Place the eggs into ice water and peel once cooled. Cut them in half.

4. Put the lettuce onto two bowls and top with the tuna mixture and eggs. Top with tomatoes and drizzle with some olive oil. Sprinkle with pepper and salt.

Turkey Salad

This recipe makes 4 servings and contains 451 calories; 33 grams fat; 28 grams protein; 6 grams net carbohydrates per serving

What You Need

For Salad

- Halved pecans, .5 c

- Raspberries, .5 pint

- Pepper

- Salt

- Crumbled goat cheese, 4 oz.

- Turkey breasts, 2

- Baby spinach, 10 oz.

For Vinaigrette

- Pepper

- Salt

- Dijon mustard, 1 tbsp.

- Raspberries .75 c

- Water, .25 c

- Olive oil, .25 c

- Vinegar, .25 c

- Chopped onion, 1

- Swerve, 1 tbsp.

What to Do

1. Place the salt, oil, onion, water, mustard, pepper, raspberries, vinegar, and swerve into a blender. Process until well blended. Press the mixture through a mesh sieve to get rid of the seeds. Set to the side.

2. Season the turkey breast with pepper and salt. Put a skillet on medium heat and place turkey into the skillet.

3. Cook eight minutes, turn over and cook another eight minutes.

4. Take the goat cheese, pecan halves, raspberries, and spinach and divide it evenly between four bowls. Slice the turkey breasts and add them to the top of the salad. Drizzle on the vinaigrette and enjoy.

Steak Salad

This recipe makes 4 servings and contains 325 calories; 19 grams fat; 28 grams protein; 4 grams net carbohydrates per serving

What You Need

For the Dressing

- Red wine vinegar, 1 tbsp.

- Pepper

- Salt

- Erythritol, 1 tsp.

- Olive oil, 3 tbsp. + extra to drizzle

- Dijon mustard, 2 tsp.

For Salad

- Pepper

- Salt

- Mixed salad greens, 2 c

- Water, .5 c

- Chopped kohlrabi, 2

- Chopped green beans, 1 c

- Sliced tomatoes, 3

- Sliced green onions, 3

- Rump steak, .5 lb., fat trimmed

What to Do

1. You need to warm your oven to 400. Put the kohlrabi on a baking sheet and coat with the oil. Put into the oven for 25 minutes.

2. Once cooked, allow it to cook.

3. Mix the olive oil, vinegar, pepper, salt, erythritol, and Dijon mustard together. Whisk to combine. Set to the side.

4. Preheat a cast iron skillet. Rub the steaks with pepper and salt. Put steaks into the skillet and sear on each side. Continue to cook until steaks are to your desired doneness. Let the steak rest for five minutes before slicing.

5. In salad bowls, add the sliced steak, greens, kohlrabi, green beans, tomatoes, and green onions. Drizzle with dressing and toss to combine.

6. Serve warm with some low carb bread if desired.

Tuna Caprese Salad

This recipe makes 4 servings and contains 360 calories; 31 grams fat; 21 grams protein; 1 gram net carbohydrates per serving

What You Need

- Juice of one lemon

- EVOO, 2 tbsp.

- Pitted and sliced black olives, .5 c

- Basil, 6 leaves

- Sliced mozzarella, 8 oz.

- Sliced tomatoes, 2

- Chunked tuna in water, 2 – 10 oz. cans, drained

What to Do

1. Put the drained tuna into the middle of a serving platter. Place the tomato slices and cheese around the tuna. Alternate a slice of cheese, tomato, and basil leaf until all the way around the platter.

2. Sprinkle the black olives on top and drizzle with lemon juice and olive oil.

Asian Beef Salad

This recipe makes 2 servings and contains 385 calories; 98 grams fat; 34 grams protein; 7 grams net carbohydrates per serving

What You Need

For Steaks

- Grated ginger, 1 tbsp.

- Olive oil, 1 tbsp.

- Chili flakes, 1 tsp.

- Fish sauce, 1 tbsp.

- Ribeye steak, .66 lb.

For Salad

- Scallions, 2

- Cherry tomatoes, 3 oz.

- Cucumber, 2

- Lettuce, 1 head

- Red onion, .5

- Cilantro

- Sesame seeds, 1 tbsp.

- For Mayo:

- Pepper

- Salt

- Lime juice, .5 tbsp.

- Olive oil, .5 c

- Sesame oil, 1 tbsp.

- Egg yolk

- Dijon mustard, 1 tsp.

What to Do

1. Make the mayo: Add the egg yolk and mustard into a bowl and whisk together. While whisking, slowly add in olive oil. You can do this by hand or using an immersion blender. After the mayo is emulsified, add in spices, sesame oil, and lime juice. Place this to the side.

2. For the steak: Mix the fish sauce, ginger, chili flakes, and olive oil together. Add to a large zip-top bag. Place ribeye into the mixture and marinate it for 15 minutes.

3. While steak is marinating, chop all vegetables for the salad except scallions. Divide these evenly between two plates

4. Place a skillet on medium heat, put the sesame seeds into the skillet and let them roast for a few minutes. Put these to the side.

5. Remove ribeye from the bag and pat dry. Place in the same skillet and sear on all sides. Continue to cook until it is done to your liking. This cut of meat is best at medium.

6. Place the scallions to the skillet and cook them for a few minutes.

7. Slice the steak thinly. Add the scallions and beef to the tops of the vegetables. Sprinkle with sesame seeds. Serve with the mayo as dressing.

Bacon and Blue Cheese Salad

This recipe makes 4 servings and contains 205 calories; 20 grams fat; 4 grams protein; 2 grams net carbohydrates per serving

What You Need

- Pepper

- Salt

- EVOO, 3 tbsp.

- White wine vinegar, 1 tbsp.

- Crumbled blue cheese, 1.5 c

- Sliced bacon, 8

- Mixed salad greens, 2 – 8 oz. bags

What to Do

1. Place the salad greens into a salad bowl. Set to the side.

2. Cook the bacon in a skillet on medium until crisp. Place on paper towels to drain. Let cool until able to crumble with hands. Once crumbled, sprinkle on top of greens. Add in half the blue cheese, and toss to combine. Set to the side.

3. In a small bowl, whisk the pepper, salt, olive, and vinegar until combined. Drizzle about half over salad, toss again, and add remaining cheese.

4. Divide into four plates and serve with more dressing if desired.

Prawn Salad

This recipe makes 4 servings and contains 215 calories; 20 grams fat; 8 grams protein; 2 grams net carbohydrates per serving

What You Need

For Dressing

- Lemon juice, 2 tbsp.

- Garlic mayonnaise, .5 c

- Dijon mustard, 1 tsp.

For Salad

- Chili Pepper

- Salt

- Peeled and deveined tiger prawns, 1 lb.

- Olive oil, 3 tbsp.

- Baby arugula, 4 c

What to Do

1. Whisk the mustard, lemon juice, and mayonnaise together. Place in the refrigerator until ready to use.

2. Place a skillet on medium and warm two tablespoons olive oil. Lay the prawns in a bowl and top with chili pepper and salt. Toss to coat. Place in the olive oil and cook until pink. Take out of skillet and place on a plate to be used later.

3. Put the arugula in a serving bowl and pour about half the dressing on top. Toss and add the rest of the dressing if desired.

4. Place the salad on four plates, top with prawns, and serve.

Garlicky Chicken Salad

This recipe makes 4 servings and contains 286 calories; 23 grams fat; 14 grams protein; 4 grams net carbohydrates per serving

What You Need

- Crumbled blue cheese, 1 c

- Red wine vinegar, 1 tbsp.

- Garlic powder, 2 tbsp.

- Mixed salad greens, 1.5 c

- Olive oil, 1 tsp.

- Pepper

- Salt

- Skinless, boneless, chicken breasts, 2

What to Do

1. Place the chicken breasts between two pieces of saran wrap. Beat the breasts with a meat mallet or rolling pin. Season with garlic powder, pepper, and salt.

2. Place a cast iron skillet on high and warm oil, fry the chicken for four minutes on both sides until golden. It needs to reach 165. Place cooked chicken on a cutting board and let cool before slicing.

3. Toss greens with red wine vinegar and divide evenly between four plates. Divide the chicken between the four salads and sprinkle with blue cheese. Serve.

Strawberry Spinach Salad

This recipe makes 2 servings and contains 445 calories; 34 grams fat; 33 grams protein; 5 grams net carbohydrates per serving

What You Need

- Pepper

- Salt

- Raspberry vinaigrette, 4 tbsp.

- Grated goat cheese, 1.5 c

- Flaked almonds, .5 c

- Sliced strawberries, 4

- Spinach, 4 c

What to Do

1. You need to warm your oven to 400. Place two pieces of parchment paper and place it on a baking sheet. Place the goat cheese into two circles. Put into the oven for ten minutes.

2. Find two bowls that are the same size and put them upside down. Carefully place the parchment on top of the bowls to form the cheese into bowls. Let sit for 15 minutes.

3. Once bowls have hardened, divide the spinach between the bowls. Drizzle the top with vinaigrette. Sprinkle on strawberries and almonds.

4. Add in the green beans, chili pepper, salt, coconut milk, and place the shrimp back into the skillet. Stir well to combine. Cook an additional four minutes. Lower heat and simmer another three minutes, occasionally stirring.

5. Adjust any seasonings that you need.

6. Ladle into bowls and serve with some cauli-rice if desired.

Warm Artichoke Salad

This recipe makes 4 servings and contains 170 calories; 13 grams fat; 1 gram protein; 5 grams net carbohydrates per serving

What You Need

- Caper brine, .25 tsp.

- Capers, 1 tbsp.

- Pepper, .25 tsp.

- Salt, .5 tsp.

- Lemon zest, .25 tsp.

- Chopped dill, 1 tbsp.

- Balsamic vinegar, 2 tsp.

- Olive oil, .25 c

- Sliced olives, .25 c

- Halved cherry peppers, .25 c

- Water, 6 c

- Baby artichokes, 6

What to Do

1. Pour the water into a pot and add salt. Place on medium.

2. Trim the artichokes and cut them in half, and add to the pot. Allow to boil.

3. Lower the heat and simmer for 20 minutes until tender.

4. Place the remaining ingredients into a bowl except for the olives. Stir well to combine.

5. Drain the artichokes and put them onto a serving plate.

6. Pour the vinaigrette over the artichokes and toss.

7. Top with sliced olives.

Spinach Bacon Salad

This recipe makes 4 servings and contains 350 calories; 33 grams fat; 7 grams protein; 3 grams net carbohydrates per serving

What You Need

For Salad

- Chopped hard-boiled eggs, 2

- Chopped lettuce, 2 small

- Spinach, 2 c

- Cooked, crumbled bacon, 4 slices

- Sliced green onion, 1

- Sliced avocado, 1

- Chopped avocado, 1

For Vinaigrette

- Dijon mustard, 1 tsp.

- Apple cider vinegar, 1 tbsp.

- Olive oil, 3 tbsp.

What to Do

1. Into a large bowl, place green onion, chopped avocado, eggs, lettuce, and spinach. Toss to combine.

2. Whisk the vinaigrette ingredients together.

3. Pour the dressing on the salad and toss again to coat.

4. Divide out into four plates and top with crumbled bacon and sliced avocados.

Crab Meat Salad

This recipe makes 4 servings and contains 182 calories; 15 grams fat; 12 grams protein; 2 grams net carbohydrates per serving

What You Need

For Salad

- Chopped dill, 1 tbsp.

- Crab meat, 2 c

- Sliced black olives, .5 c

- Diced celery, .33 c

- Cauliflower, 5 c

For Dressing

- Salt

- Swerve, 2 tsp.

- Lemon juice, 2 tbsp.

- Pepper

- Celery seeds, .25 tsp.

- Apple cider vinegar, 1 tsp.

- Mayonnaise, .5 c

What to Do

1. Put the dill, shrimp, celery, and cauliflower into a large bowl.

2. In a small bowl, add the lemon juice, sweetener, celery seeds, vinegar, and mayonnaise. Whisk to combine. Sprinkle with salt. Do a taste test and adjust if needed.

3. Pour over salad and toss to combine.

4. Place into the refrigerator for at least one hour.

5. Divide into four plates and top with olives.

Treats

Cinnamon Smoothie

This recipe makes 2 servings and contains 492 calories; 47 grams fat; 18 grams protein; 6 grams net carbohydrates per serving

What You Need

- Coconut milk, 2 c

- Vanilla, .5 tsp.

- Cinnamon, 1 tsp.

- Liquid stevia, 5 drops

- Vanilla protein powder, 1 tsp.

What to Do

1. Simply add everything to your blender and mix until it forms a smooth consistency

2. Divide into two glasses and enjoy.

Blueberry Smoothie

This recipe makes 2 servings and contains 353 calories; 32 grams fat; 15 grams protein; 6 grams net carbohydrates per serving

What You Need

- Spinach, 1 c
- Coconut milk, 1 c
- Mint, 4 sprigs – garnish
- Ice cubes, 4
- Coconut oil, 2 tbsp.
- Plain protein powder, 1 tsp.
- Blueberries, .5 c
- Chopped English cucumber, .5

What to Do

1. Simply add everything to your blender, except for the mint, and mix until it forms a smooth consistency.

2. Divide into two glasses and garnish with mint.

Vanilla Ice Cream

This recipe makes 1 serving, and contains 238 calories; 22 grams fat; 5 grams protein; 2 grams net carbohydrates per serving

What You Need

- Vanilla, 1 tbsp.

- Heavy cream, 1.25 c

- Erythritol, .5 c

- Cream of tartar, .25 tsp.

- Eggs, 4

What to Do

1. Separate the eggs. Beat the cream of tartar into the egg whites. As the egg whites start to thicken up, mix in the erythritol. Continue to whisk the eggs whites until they form stiff peaks.

2. Using a different bowl, beat the cream. Whisk until it forms soft peaks form. Make sure that you don't overbeat the whipping cream.

3. In another bowl, mix the vanilla and the egg yolks.

4. Carefully fold the whipped cream and egg whites together.

5. Carefully fold the egg yolk mixture into everything. You don't want to cause the mixture to fall, but you want to make sure everything is well mixed.

6. Pour this into a loaf pan and freeze for at least two hours. Let it sit at room temp for a few minutes to make it easier to scoop out.

Brownies

This recipe makes 16 servings and contains 136 calories; 12 grams fat; 1 gram protein; 4 grams net carbohydrates per serving

What You Need

- Salt, .25 tsp.

- Baking powder, .5 tsp.

- Unsweetened cocoa powder, 100 g

- Powdered erythritol, 170 g

- Eggs, 3

- Almond butter, 1 c

What to Do

1. Start by placing your oven to 325.

2. Mix together the erythritol and almond butter using a food processor.

3. Add in the salt, baking powder, cocoa powder, and eggs. Blend everything together until smooth.

4. Grease a square baking dish and pour into the prepared baking dish. Bake for 12 minutes.

5. Allow the brownies to cool for 30 minutes before slicing it into 16 squares. Enjoy.

Pecan Peanut Butter Bars

This recipe makes 12 servings and contains 225 calories; 22 grams fat; 2 grams protein; 4 grams net carbohydrates per serving

What You Need

- Vanilla, 1 tsp.

- Peanut butter, .5 c

- Coconut oil, .5 c

- Pecans, 2 c

What to Do

1. Grease a casserole dish and spread the pecans in the bottom of the dish.

2. Add the oil and peanut butter to a microwavable bowl. Microwave it for 30 seconds. Whisk, and continue until everything has melted together.

3. Add in the vanilla.

4. Top the pecans with the mixture. Refrigerate this for about an hour or until set.

Peanut Butter Cookie

This recipe makes 12 servings and contains 80 calories; 5 grams fat; 2 grams protein; 6 grams net carbohydrates per serving

What You Need

- Egg, 1

- Powdered erythritol, .5 c

- Peanut butter, 1 c

What to Do

1. Start by placing the oven to 350.

2. Stir everything together.

3. Line a baking sheet with parchment and form 1-inch balls of dough, laying them on the baking sheet.

4. Press the cookies down with a fork.

5. Bake for 12 minutes.

6. Allow them to cook for five minutes before serving.

Strawberry Butter

This recipe makes 48 servings and contains 23 calories; 2 grams fat; 0 gram protein; 1 gram net carbohydrates per serving

What You Need

- Vanilla, 1 tsp.

- Lemon juice, .5 tbsp.

- Shredded unsweetened coconut, 2 c

- Strawberries, .75 c

- Coconut oil, 1 tbsp.

What You Need

1. Add the coconut to your food processor and mix until it forms a paste. This is going to take around 15 minutes.

2. Add in the coconut oil, strawberries, lemon juice, and vanilla into the coconut puree. Process everything together until it becomes smooth. You may want to scrape the sides of the processor down from time to time.

3. Pour this through a fine mesh sieve to get rid of the strawberry seeds if you want a smooth consistency. Using the back of the spoon can help you to push everything through.

4. Pour into an airtight container and then refrigerate. It will need to be kept in the refrigerator. This will last for two weeks.

Peanut Butter Mousse

This recipe makes 4 servings and contains 280 calories; 28 grams fat; 6 grams protein; 3 grams net carbohydrates per serving

What You Need

- Heavy cream, 1 c

- Peanut butter, .25 c

- Vanilla, 1 tsp.

- Liquid stevia, 4 drops

What to Do

1. Add everything to a bowl and beat together until it forms stiff peaks. This will take about five minutes. If you have a stand mixer, it will be easier on your hand.

2. Spoon into four individual servings bowls and refrigerate for 30 minutes before servings.

Peanut Butter Cups

This recipe makes 6 servings and contains 231 calories; 15 grams fat; 2 grams protein; 3 grams net carbohydrates per serving

What You Need

- Vanilla, .25 tsp.

- Stevia, .5 tsp.

- Cocoa powder, 1 tbsp.

- Unsweetened baker's chocolate, 1 oz.

- Coconut oil, .25 c

- Peanut butter, .25 c

What to Do

1. Add the chocolate to a pot and let it melt. Make sure you watch the chocolate close so that it doesn't burn.

2. Stir in the peanut butter. The softer your peanut butter is, the easier it will be to mix in. Mix in the coconut oil and cocoa powder next, stirring until completely mixed.

3. You can use silicone molds or paper-lined cupcake tins. Pour the chocolate mixture into the cupcake molds.

4. Place this in the freezer and let it set up until solid. This will take about an hour. Once they have been set up, you can remove them from the molds and keep them stored in an airtight container. You can also leave them in the molds if you would like. They should be kept in the refrigerator.

Mound Bars

This recipe makes 16 servings and contains 43 calories; 5 grams fat; 1 gram protein; 1 gram net carbohydrates per serving

What You Need

- Coconut oil, .33 c

- Shredded unsweetened coconut, .25 c

- Unsweetened cocoa powder, .25 c

- Salt

- Liquid stevia, 4 drops

What to Do

1. Line a 6-inch square casserole dish with some parchment paper and set to the side.

2. Add the coconut oil, salt, cocoa, and Stevie to a pot. Mix everything together until melted and combined. This will take about three minutes.

3. Stir in the coconut and then press the mixture into the prepared casserole dish.

4. Refrigerate the bars until they are hardened. This will take about 30 minutes.

5. Once they are set, slice into 16 pieces and keep them stored in a cool place and in an airtight container.

Peppermint Mocha Drops

This recipe makes 6 servings and contains 183 calories; 19 grams fat; 0 gram protein; 3 grams net carbohydrates per serving

What You Need

- Softened coconut oil, .25 c

- Vanilla, .5 tsp.

- Softened butter, .25 c

- Peppermint extract, 2 tsp.

- Melted dark chocolate, .33 c

- Liquid stevia, 40 drops

What to Do

1. Simply place everything in a blender and combine until it forms a smooth mixture.

2. Using six small silicon baking cups, scoop two tablespoons of the mixture into the cups.

3. Place these molds in the freezer until they become hard. This will take about 15 minutes. Keep them stored in the refrigerator or in the freezer.

4. When you are ready to use them, add a drop to a blender along with a cup of coffee and blend until smooth.

Mocha Bonbons

This recipe makes 15 servings and contains 112 calories; 13 grams fat; 6 grams protein; 3 grams net carbohydrates per serving

What You Need

- Softened cream cheese, 8 oz.

- Coffee beans, 15 pieces

- Strong coffee, .25 c

- Cocoa butter, 2 tbsp.

- Truvia, .25 c

- MCT oil, 3 tbsp.

- Cocoa, 2 tbsp.

- Dark chocolate chips, .66 c

What to Do

1. Place the softened cream cheese, cocoa, sweetener, and coffee in a stand mixer. Slowly increase the speed of the mixer; you don't want to sling the coffee everywhere. Continue to mix until the mixture is combined and fluffy. Chill the cream cheese mixture for four hours, or overnight.

2. Using a small cookie scoop, scoop out the mixture into 15 balls onto wax paper. Allow the balls to freeze for half an hour.

3. Melt together the MCT oil, cocoa butter, and chocolate in the microwave. Be careful not to let the chocolate burn.

4. Cover the truffles with the chocolate and press a coffee bean into the top of each truffle. Freeze for an hour and keep stored in an airtight container.

Herb Crusted Goat Cheese

This recipe makes 4 servings and contains 304 calories; 28 grams fat; 12 grams protein; 2 grams net carbohydrates per serving

What You Need

- Chopped parsley, 1 tbsp.

- Goat cheese log, 8 oz.

- Chopped oregano, 1 tbsp.

- Pepper

- Chopped thyme, 1 tsp.

- Chopped walnuts, 6 oz.

What to Do

2. Put the pepper, thyme, parsley, oregano, and walnuts into a food processor and pulse until everything is chopped fine.

3. Place this mixture onto a plate. Gently roll the cheese log in the walnuts. Press slightly to adhere the walnuts onto the cheese.

4. Slice and enjoy.

Coconut Chips

This recipe makes 4 servings and contains 261 calories; 27 grams fat; 2.3 grams protein; 3 grams net carbohydrates per serving

What You Need

- Desiccated coconut, 2 cups

- Curry powder, 1 tsp.

- Salt, .5 tsp.

- Cayenne, .25 tsp.

- Garlic powder, 1 tsp.

- Melted EVOO, 2 tbsp.

What to Do

1. You need to warm your oven to 350. Line a cooking sheet with parchment.

2. Place the coconut, salt, spices, and coconut oil into a bowl. Stir to combine.

3. Spread coconut onto the prepared baking sheet and bake for five minutes.

4. Carefully take out of the oven and let cool completely.

Cashew Bars

This recipe makes 2 servings and contains 190 calories; 18 grams fat; 4 grams protein; 2 grams net carbohydrates per serving

What You Need

- Salt

- Cinnamon, 1 tsp.

- Melted butter, .25 c

- Shredded coconut, .25 c

- Maple syrup, .25 c

- Cashews, .5 c

- Almond flour, 1 c

What to Do

1. Place a sheet of parchment paper onto a baking sheet.

2. Place the melted butter and almond flour into a bowl. Add in the salt, cinnamon, maple syrup, and shredded coconut. Stir well to combine.

3. Chop one-half cup of the cashews and add these to the dough.

4. Spread dough onto the prepared baking sheet.

5. Put into the refrigerator and leave for three hours.

6. Cut evenly into bars and enjoy.

Pizza Chips

This recipe makes 8 servings and contains 250 calories; 19 grams fat; 16 grams protein; 3 grams net carbohydrates per serving

What You Need

- Italian seasoning, 2 tsp.

- Shredded Parmesan, 8 oz.

- Shredded mozzarella, 8 oz.

- Sliced pepperoni, 10 oz.

What to Do

1. You need to warm your oven to 400.

2. Take two baking sheets and line them with aluminum foil.

3. Place the pepperoni evenly in one layer onto the prepared baking sheet.

4. Sprinkle each piece with Italian seasoning, parmesan, and mozzarella.

5. Put into the oven for ten minutes.

6. Take out of the oven and allow to cool for five minutes or until they have turned crispy.

7. If you want to, you can dip these in marinara.

Coconut Candy

This recipe makes 10 servings and contains 104 calories; 11 grams fat; 0 gram protein; 1 gram net carbohydrates per serving

What You Need

- Sweetener, 1 tsp.

- Unsweetened shredded coconut, 1 oz.

- Melted coconut oil, .33 c

- Softened coconut butter, .33 c

What to Do

1. Mix everything together until the sweetener is dissolved and everything is well combined.

2. Pour into silicone molds or a cupcake tin that has been lined with paper liners. Refrigerate for one hour.

3. Keep stored in the refrigerator in an airtight container.

Chocolate Mint Fat Bombs

This recipe makes 6 servings and contains 161 calories; 19 grams fat; 0 gram protein; 1 gram net carbohydrates per serving

What You Need

- Peppermint extract, .5 tsp.

- Melted coconut oil, .5 c

- Sweetener, 1 tbsp.

- Cocoa powder, 2 tbsp.

What to Do

1. Add the sweetener and peppermint extract to the melted coconut oil.

2. Pour half of this mixture into another bowl along with the cocoa powder.

3. Place paper liners into a cupcake tin and pour half of the chocolate mixture into the liners. Put this in the refrigerator and leave for ten minutes.

4. Remove from the chocolate out of the fridge and pour in the mint mixture. Refrigerate for another ten minutes.

5. Take out of the refrigerator and pour the rest of the chocolate on top. Refrigerate once again to let this layer harden.

6. Unmold and enjoy.

7. Keep these refrigerated.

Mini Strawberry Cheesecakes

This recipe makes 8 servings and contains 129 calories; 13 grams fat; 2 grams protein; 2 grams net carbohydrates per serving

What You Need

- Vanilla, 1 tsp.

- Liquid stevia, 10 to 15 drops

- Softened coconut oil, .25 c

- Softened cream cheese, .75 c

- Mashed strawberries, .5 c

What to Do

1. Mix everything together with a hand mixer. You could also do this with a blender.

2. Take a mini muffin tin and place paper liners into each one. Carefully fill each cup with mixture.

3. Place in the freezer. Let freeze for two hours.

4. These should be kept in the refrigerator.

Avocado Crunch Bombs

This recipe makes 8 servings and contains 151 calories; 14 grams fat; 3 grams protein; 5 grams net carbohydrates per serving

What You Need

- Sliced bacon, 4

- Avocados, 2

- Pecans, 6

What to Do

1. Place a skillet on top of the stove on medium heat until crispy. Drain the bacon.

2. Allow to cool. When cooled, crumble bacon.

3. Slice the avocados in half lengthwise, open and carefully remove the pit. Spoon out the flesh and place into a bowl. Mash well. Add some lemon or lime juice to keep avocados from oxidizing.

4. You can either chop the pecans with a knife or put them into a food processor and pulse until chopped.

5. Place the bacon and pecans into the mashed avocados. Mix well until everything is thoroughly incorporated.

6. Use a small ice cream scoop to make balls.

7. Keep refrigerated.

Pumpkin Mug Cake

This recipe makes 1 serving, and contains 385 calories; 31 grams fat; 14 grams protein; 3 grams net carbohydrates per serving

What You Need

- Liquid stevia, 5 to 10 drops

- Baking soda, pinch

- Pumpkin puree, 2 tbsp.

- Pumpkin spice mix, .5 tsp.

- Erythritol, 2 tbsp.

- Egg, 1

- Ground chia seeds, 1 tbsp.

- Almond flour, 2 tbsp.

- Coconut oil, 1 tbsp.

- Coconut flour, 1 tbsp.

What to Do

1. Put all the ingredients into a microwave safe mug. Stir well to combine. Microwave for two minutes on high.

Snacks and Sides

Bacon Deviled Eggs

This recipe makes 12 servings and contains 85 calories; 7 grams fat; 6 grams protein; 2 grams net carbohydrates per serving

What You Need

- Cooked, chopped bacon, 6 slices

- Pepper

- Dijon, .5 tsp.

- Shredded Swiss cheese, .25 c

- Chopped avocado, .25

- Mayonnaise, .25 c

- Hardboiled eggs, 6

What to Do

1. Slice the eggs in half lengthwise.

2. Carefully take the yolks out and place them in a bowl. Lay the whites on a plate with the hollow-side up.

3. Break the yolks apart with a fork and mix in the Dijon, cheese, avocado, and mayonnaise. Season with a bit of pepper.

4. Spoon the yolks into the egg whites and top with some crumbled bacon. Enjoy.

Parmesan Chips

This recipe makes 4 servings and contains 227 calories; 16 grams fat; 13 grams protein; 7 grams net carbohydrates per serving

What You Need

- Garlic powder, .5 tsp.

- Rosemary, 1 tsp.

- Almond flour, 4 tbsp.

- Grated parmesan, 6 oz.

What to Do

1. Start by placing your oven to 350.

2. Combine the almond flour and parmesan cheese together. Mix in the garlic powder and rosemary. Mix until everything is well combined.

3. Line a baking sheet with parchment, and place tablespoon size circles of the cheese mixture.

4. Bake for 10-15 minutes.

5. Allow the chips to cool before servings.

Kale Chips

This recipe makes 2 servings and contains 107 calories; 7 grams fat; 4 grams protein; 5 grams net carbohydrates per serving

What You Need

- Pepper

- Salt

- Kale leaves, 12 pieces

- Olive oil, 3 tsp.

What to Do

1. Start by placing your oven to 350.

2. Lay some parchment on a cooking sheet.

3. Wash the kale and thoroughly dry. Lay them out on the baking sheet. Drizzle them with the oil and top with pepper and salt.

4. Bake the chips for 10-15 minutes. Enjoy.

Bacon Fat Bombs

This recipe makes 12 servings and contains 89 calories; 8 grams fat; 3 grams protein; 0 gram net carbohydrates per serving

What You Need

- Room temp cream cheese, 2 oz.

- Room temp goat cheese, 2 oz.

- Pepper

- Chopped, cooked bacon, 8 slices

- Room temp, butter, .25 c

What to Do

1. Place parchment on a baking sheet and set to the side.

2. Mix together the pepper, bacon, butter, cream cheese, and goat cheese in a bowl until well combined.

3. Place tablespoon size mounds on the baking sheet and place in the freezer until they are firm but not completely frozen. This will take about an hour.

4. These will keep in an airtight container for about two weeks.

Golden Rosti

This recipe makes 8 servings and contains 171 calories; 15 grams fat; 5 grams protein; 3 grams net carbohydrates per serving

What You Need

- Butter, 2 tbsp.

- Minced garlic, 2 tsp.

- Chopped bacon, 8 slices

- Pepper

- Shredded acorn squash, 1 c

- Salt

- Shredded celeriac, 1 c

- Chopped thyme, 1 tsp.

- Grated parmesan, 2 tbsp.

What to Do

1. Add the bacon to a large skillet and cook until crispy.

2. While the bacon is cooking, mix together the squash, thyme, celeriac, garlic, and parmesan. Add in a generous amount of pepper and salt. Place this to the side.

3. Drain the bacon. Once cooled, break the bacon into the rosti mixture. Mix everything together.

4. Reserve two tablespoons of the bacon fat, add to the skillet along with the butter.

5. Resume the heat and add in the rosti mixture and spread it around to create a large patty that is around an inch thick.

6. Cook the rosti until it has browned on the bottom and crisped up.

7. Flip over and then cook it on the others until it has crisped up and is cooked all the way through.

8. Remove from the pan and then slice it into eight equal pieces.

Broccoli Cheddar Tots

This recipe makes 2 servings and contains 319 calories; 22 grams fat; 21 grams protein; 7 grams net carbohydrates per serving

What You Need

- Broccoli florets, 2 c

- Cooking spray

- Eggs, 2

- Salt, 1 tsp.

- Sharp cheddar cheese, .5 c

- Almond flour, .25 c

- Parmesan, .25 c

- Coconut flour, 2 tbsp.

- Diced onion, .25 c

What to Do

1. Start by placing your oven to 400. Place some parchment on a baking sheet.

2. Add the broccoli to a microwavable bowl and cover it with a damp towel. Microwave the broccoli for two minutes.

3. Remove the broccoli from the bowl and finely chop it. Add it back to the bowl and add in all of the remaining ingredients. Stir everything together until well combined.

4. Using a tablespoon, scoop out the broccoli mixture and form them into tot shapes.

5. Lay them on the baking sheet. Continue doing this until you have used all of the broccoli mixtures. Spritz the tops of the tots with the cooking spray and bake them for six minutes. Flip the tots and bake for another seven minutes.

Pecorino Mushroom Burgers

This recipe makes 4 servings and contains 370 calories; 30 grams fat; 16 grams protein; 8 grams net carbohydrates per serving

What You Need

- Pecorino cheese, .5 c

- Whisked eggs, 2

- Mustard, 1 tsp.

- Cajun seasoning, 1 tbsp.

- Sunflower seeds, 4 tbsp.

- Hemp seeds, 4 tbsp.

- Ground flax seeds, 4 tbsp.

- Almond flour, 4 tbsp.

- Chopped Portobello mushrooms, 2 c

- Minced garlic, 2 cloves

- Softened butter, 2 tbsp.

What to Do

1. Add a tablespoon of butter to a skillet and melt. Once melted, add in the garlic and mushrooms, cooking until all of the water has cooked out of the mushrooms.

2. Add the Cajun seasoning, flax seeds, sunflower seeds, eggs, mustard, hemp seeds, almond flour, cooked mushrooms, onions, and pecorino in a bowl and mix together. Form the mixture into four patties.

3. Add the rest of the butter to a skillet and fry up the patties for seven minutes, flip, and cook them for another six minutes. Serve warm.

Roasted String Beans

This recipe makes 4 servings and contains 121 calories; 2 grams fat; 6 grams protein; 6 grams net carbohydrates per serving

What You Need

- Pepper

- Salt

- Dried thyme, .5 tsp.

- Julienned shallots, 3

- Olive oil, 3 tbsp.

- Minced garlic, 2 cloves

- Quartered tomatoes, 3

- Quartered cremini mushrooms, 1 lb.

- Halved string beans, 2 c

What to Do

1. Start by placing your oven to 450.

2. Mix together the pepper, salt, thyme, shallots, olive oil, garlic, tomatoes, mushrooms, and string beans. Spread the vegetables out on a baking sheet. Make sure that the veggies are in a single layer.

3. Bake the vegetables for 20-25 minutes. You can flip the veggies over halfway through the cooking process if you would like to. Enjoy.

Fries and Aioli

This recipe makes 4 servings and contains 205 calories; 4 grams fat; 2 grams protein; 4 grams net carbohydrates per serving

What You Need

Aioli

- Lemon juice, 3 tbsp.
- Pepper
- Salt
- Minced garlic, 2 cloves
- Mayonnaise, 4 tbsp.

Fries

- Pepper
- Salt
- Chopped parsley, 5 tbsp.
- Olive oil, 2 tbsp.
- Julienned carrots, 3
- Julienned parsnips, 6

What to Do

1. Start by placing your oven to 400.
2. Whisk together all of the aioli ingredients together and allow the mixture to refrigerate for at least 30 minutes.

3. Lay the carrots and parsnips out on a cooking sheet and drizzle them with oil. Sprinkle on the pepper and salt. Move the veggies around in the baking sheet to make sure that they are all evenly coated.

4. Bake them for 35 minutes.

5. Transfer the fries to a plate and garnish with the parsley. Serve them with aioli.

Garlic Mashed Celeriac

This recipe makes 4 servings and contains 94 calories; 0 gram fat; 2 grams protein; 6 grams net carbohydrates per serving

What You Need

- Pepper

- Salt

- Dried basil, 2 tsp.

- Garlic powder, .5 tsp.

- Sour cream, .33 c

- Butter, 2 tbsp.

- Cream cheese, 2 oz.

- Water, 4 c

- Chopped celeriac, 2 lb.

What to Do

1. Add the celeriac to a pot of water and boil. Let this cook for 5 minutes and then turn the heat down and let the celeriac simmer for about 15 minutes. Drain out the water.

2. Put the cooked celeriac in a bowl with the pepper, salt, basil, garlic powder, sour cream, butter, and cream cheese. Use an electric mixer on medium speed to mix everything together and to create a creamy consistency. This is perfect served with grilled salmon.

Spicy Deviled Eggs

This recipe makes 12 servings and contains 112 calories; 9 grams fat; 6 grams protein; 0 gram net carbohydrates per serving

What You Need

- Ice water bath

- Chopped parsley – garnish

- Pinch of paprika

- Dijon, .25 tsp.

- Worcestershire sauce, .5 tsp.

- Mixed dried herbs, 1 tsp.

- Chili pepper

- Salt

- Mayonnaise, 6 tbsp.

- Water, 1.5 c

- Eggs, 12

What to Do

1. Bring a pot of water to a boil. Slowly and carefully ease the eggs into the boiling water. Allow them to cook for 12 minutes.

2. Once the eggs have cooked, drain off the hot water and place the eggs directly in an ice water bath to cool off.

3. Once you can handle the eggs, peel them.

4. Slice the eggs lengthwise and carefully pop the yolks out and place them in a bowl. Set the whites on a plate with the hollow side up.

5. Break the yolks up with a fork. Add in the paprika, mustard, Worcestershire sauce, dried herbs, chili pepper, salt, and mayonnaise. Mix everything together until it forms a smooth paste.

6. Spoon the mixture into the egg whites. If you want to make them look pretty, you can also add the yolk mixture to a piping bag and pip in rosettes.

7. Garnish the top of the deviled eggs with parsley and enjoy.

Avocado Crostini

This recipe makes 4 servings and contains 195 calories; 12 grams fat; 13 grams protein; 3 grams net carbohydrates per serving

What You Need

- Chia seeds, 1 tbsp.

- Lemon juice, 1 tsp.

- Chopped raw walnuts, .33 c

- Coconut oil, 1.5 tbsp.

- Salt, .33 tsp.

- Mashed avocado, 1 c

- Nori sheets, 4

- Low-carb baguette, 8 slices

What to Do

1. Flake the nori sheets apart into small pieces and place in a bowl.

2. In a separate bowl, mix together the lemon juice, salt, and avocado. Mix in the nori flakes and set to the side.

3. Lay the baguette slices out on a baking sheet and toast them under the broiler for about two minutes. Make sure the bread doesn't burn.

4. Take them out of the oven and brush the coconut oil on both sides of the baguette slices.

5. Top the crostini with the avocado mixture and top with the walnuts and chia seeds. Enjoy.

Low-Carb Cheddar Bay Biscuits

This recipe makes 6-8 servings and contains 153 calories; 14 grams fat; 5 grams protein; 1 gram net carbohydrates per serving

What You Need

- Greek yogurt, .33 c

- Grated sharp cheddar cheese, 1.25 c

- Melted butter, .33 c

- Eggs, 5

- Baking powder, 1 tsp.

- Salt

- Garlic powder, 2 tsp.

- Almond flour, .33 c

What to Do

1. Start by placing your oven to 350.

2. Mix together the cheddar cheese, baking powder, salt, garlic powder, and almond flour.

3. Mix the yogurt, butter, and eggs together in another bowl. Add the yogurt mixture into the almond flour mixture. Stir everything together until it forms a biscuit-like consistency.

4. Drop biscuits sized dollops of the biscuit dough onto a baking sheet. Make sure that you keep them about two inches apart.

5. Bake the biscuits for 12 minutes, or until they are golden brown on top. Enjoy.

Spinach and Cheese Balls

This recipe makes 8 servings and contains 160 calories; 15 grams fat; 8 grams protein; 1 gram net carbohydrates per serving

What You Need

- Almond flour, 1 c

- Spinach, 8 oz.

- Eggs, 2

- Garlic powder, 1 tsp.

- Parmesan, .33 c

- Melted butter, 2 tbsp.

- Onion powder, 1 tbsp.

- Heavy cream, 3 tbsp.

- Pepper, .25 tsp.

- Nutmeg, .25 tsp.

- Ricotta cheese, .33 c

What to Do

1. Simply add the ingredients to a blender. Mix everything together until it forms a smooth mixture.

2. Pour the mixture into a bowl and freeze for about ten minutes to firm it up slightly.

3. Set your oven to 350.

4. Once firm, form the mixture into balls and lay them out on a parchment-lined baking sheet.

5. Bake the cheese balls for 10-12 minutes. Once browned, enjoy or store in an airtight container once cooled and keep refrigerated.

Stuffed Piquillo Peppers

This recipe makes 8 servings and contains 132 calories; 11 grams fat; 6 grams protein; 3 grams net carbohydrates per serving

What You Need

- Balsamic vinegar, 1 tbsp.

- Prosciutto, 4 slices – sliced in half

- Olive oil, 1 tbsp.

- Roasted piquillo peppers, 8

Filling

- Chopped mint, 1 tbsp.

- Minced garlic, .5 tsp.

- Chopped parsley, 3 tbsp.

- Olive oil, 1 tbsp.

- Heavy cream, 3 tbsp.

- Goat cheese, 8 oz.

What to Do

1. Mix the filling ingredients together. Add the filling to a freezer bag and push the mixture to the corner of the bag. Trim off the corner.

2. Take the peppers and clean out the inside. Add about two tablespoons of the filling mixture into each of the peppers.

3. Wrap a slice of prosciutto around each of the peppers. Secure the prosciutto with toothpicks.

4. Place them on a plate and top with a drizzle of balsamic vinegar and olive oil.

Coconut Ginger Macaroons

This recipe makes 6 servings and contains 97 calories; 3 grams fat; 6 grams protein; 0 gram net carbohydrates per serving

What You Need

- Water, 1 c

- Pinch of chili powder

- Swerve, .25 c

- Finely shredded coconut, 1 c

- Egg whites, 6

- Pureed ginger root, 2 fingers

What to Do

1. Start by place the oven to 350.

2. Lay some parchment on a cooking sheet.

3. In a heat-safe bowl, mix together the chili powder, swerve, shredded coconut, egg whites, and ginger.

4. Boil a pot of water. Make sure that the bowl with the coconut mixture can fit over the pot of water with the bottom touching the water.

5. Set the bowl over the boiling water and continue to whisk the mixture until it becomes glossy. This will take about four minutes.

6. Place the mixture in a piping bag fitted and pipe out around 40-50 macaroons onto your prepared baking sheet. Cook these for about 15 minutes or until browned.

7. Once the macaroons are cooked, place them on a wire rack to cool. You can garnish them with some angel hair chili if you want.

Chicken Fritters with Dip

This recipe makes 4 servings and contains 151 calories; 7 grams fat; 12 grams protein; 1 gram net carbohydrates per serving

What You Need

- Finely chopped onion, 2 tbsp.

- Garlic powder, 1 tsp.

- Chopped dill, 4 tbsp. – divided

- Chopped parsley, 1 tbsp.

- Mayonnaise, 1.25 c – divided

- Olive oil, 3 tbsp.

- Grated mozzarella, 1 c

- Pepper

- Salt

- Sour cream, 1 c

- Eggs, 2

- Coconut flour, .25 c

- Thinly sliced and chopped chicken breasts, 1 lb.

What to Do

1. Mix together a cup of mayonnaise, the garlic powder, sour cream, salt, onion, parsley, and three tablespoons of dill. Cover this with saran wrap and refrigerate as you fix everything else.

2. Next, mix together the rest of the dill and mayonnaise, along with the mozzarella, pepper, salt, eggs, and coconut flour. Mix in the chicken, making sure that everything is well combined. Cover up the bowl and let the chicken marinate for at least two hours.

3. Add some olive oil to a pan and heat it up. Scoop out two tablespoons of the batter and place them in the heated pan. Use your spatula to flatten the mixture out into a fritter shape.

4. Let the mixture cook for four minutes on one side. Make sure the first side is very well browned and golden so that it holds together when you flip it.

5. Flip the fritter, cooking for another four minutes, or until completely cooked. Set the fritter onto a wire race and continue with the rest of the batter. Add extra oil as you need to.

6. Garnish the fritters with some parsley and serve with the dill dip you made earlier.

Amaretti Biscuits

This recipe makes 6 servings and contains 165 calories; 13 grams fat; 9 grams protein; 3 grams net carbohydrates per serving

What You Need

- Powdered swerve, .75 c – topping

- Softened butter, .25 c

- Mascarpone cheese, .25 c

- Amaretto whiskey, 7 tbsp.

- Juice of a lemon

- Ground almonds, .25 c

- Pinch of salt

- Powdered swerve, 8 oz.

- Vanilla bean paste, 1 tsp.

- Beaten egg yolk

- Egg whites, 6

What to Do

1. Start by placing your oven on 300 and place some parchment paper on a baking sheet.

2. Beat together the vanilla paste, salt, and egg whites using an electric mixer. As you are mixing the egg whites, slowly add in the 8 ounces of the powdered Swerve. Keep mixing until the egg whites form stiff peaks.

3. Mix together the amaretto, lemon juice, egg yolk, and ground almonds. Carefully fold this mixture into the egg whites.

4. Add the batter to a piping bag and form 40-50 mounds onto your prepared baking sheet. Bake the biscuits for 15 minutes. They should be golden brown.

5. Whisk together the remaining swerve, butter, and mascarpone cheese. Set to the side.

6. Once the biscuits are cooked through, move them to a wire rack and allow them to cool. Place some of the mascarpone cheese mixtures onto half of the biscuits, on the flat side. Press another biscuit onto each, forming a sandwich. Sift on some extra powdered swerve if desired.

Pesto Parmesan Dip

This recipe makes 6 servings and contains 161 calories; 14 grams fat; 5 grams protein; 3 grams net carbohydrates per serving

What You Need

- Pepper

- Salt

- Sliced olives, 8

- Grated parmesan cheese, .5 c

- Pesto, 2 tbsp.

- Cream cheese, 1 c

What to Do

1. Mix all of the ingredients together

2. Place into the refrigerator for 20 minutes.

3. Keep refrigerated.

Bacon Dip

This recipe makes 12 servings and contains 190 calories; 17 grams fat; 7 grams protein; 4 grams net carbohydrates per serving

What You Need

- Sliced scallions, 1 c

- Shredded cheddar, 1 c

- Cream cheese, 1 c

- Sour cream, 1.5 c

- Sliced bacon, 5

What to Do

1. You need to warm your oven to 400.

2. Cook the bacon until crispy. Drain the cooked bacon. Once cooled, crumble.

3. Place bacon along with all the other ingredients into a mixing bowl. Combine everything together.

4. Pour into a baking dish.

5. Bake for 30 minutes.

6. Allow to cool for ten minutes before serving.

Cheddar Chips

This recipe makes 4 servings and contains 457 calories; 38 grams fat; 28 grams protein; 1 gram net carbohydrates per serving

What You Need

- Shredded cheddar, 4 c

- Salt

What to Do

1. You need to warm your oven to 350.

2. Lay a sheet of parchment paper on a cooking sheet.

3. Spoon the cheese into mounds onto the prepared baking sheet.

4. Place in the oven for five minutes. Check frequently until cheese is browned. Don't let it burn.

5. Sprinkle the cheese with salt.

6. Allow to cool completely.

Nachos

This recipe makes 2 to 4 servings and contains 599 calories; 45 grams fat; 41 grams protein; 5 grams net carbohydrates per serving

What You Need

- Shredded cheddar, 2 c

- Pork rinds, 1.5 oz. bag

- Pepper

- Chopped cilantro, 1 tbsp.

- Salt

- Lime juice, 1.5 tsp.

- Minced jalapeno, 1

- Minced garlic, 1 tsp.

- Chopped onion, .25

- Chopped tomato, 1 medium

What to Do

1. Place the tomato, onion, cilantro, jalapeno, garlic, and lime juice into a bowl. Sprinkle with pepper and salt. Stir well to combine. Set to the side for one hour.

2. You need to warm your oven to 350. Place aluminum foil onto a rimmed baking sheet.

3. Place the pork rinds in one layer onto the prepared baking sheet. Sprinkle cheese on top and then spoon on the salsa.

4. Place into the oven for 15 minutes. Remove carefully. Place onto a serving platter and enjoy.

Queso

This recipe makes 6 servings and contains 213 calories; 19 grams fat; 10 grams protein; 2 grams net carbohydrates per serving

What You Need

- Cayenne pepper, .25 tsp.

- Shredded cheddar, 6 oz.

- Goat cheese, 2 oz.

- Onion powder, .5 tsp.

- Minced garlic, 1 tsp.

- Diced, seeded, jalapeno, .5

- Coconut milk, .5 cup

What to Do

1. Place the onion powder, garlic, jalapeno, and coconut milk into a saucepan. Stir to combine.

2. Bring everything to a simmer. Add in goat cheese and whisk until completely smooth.

3. Place the cayenne and cheddar into the pan and continue to whisk until thickened.

4. Serve with vegetables or keto-friendly crackers.

Parmesan Crackers

This recipe makes 8 servings and contains 133 calories; 11 grams fat; 11 grams protein; 1 gram net carbohydrates per serving

What You Need

- Grated Parmesan cheese, 8 oz.

- Butter, 1 tsp.

What to Do

1. You need to warm your oven to 450.

2. Line a cooking sheet with parchment. Grease with one teaspoon of butter.

3. Put the Parmesan cheese on the baking sheet in mounds placed evenly apart.

4. Bake until edges have browned, around five minutes.

5. Take out of the oven and gently use a spatula to place them on paper towels. Blot any excess grease from the tops with paper towels. Let them completely cool.

Asparagus and Walnuts

This recipe makes 4 servings and contains 124 calories; 12 grams fat; 3 grams protein; 2 grams net carbohydrates per serving

What You Need

- Chopped walnuts, .25 c
- Pepper
- Salt
- Trimmed asparagus, .75 lb.
- Olive oil, 1.5 tbsp.

What to Do

1. Place a large skillet on top of the stove and warm the olive oil on medium heat.
2. Cook the asparagus until tender and slightly browned. This will take about five minutes.
3. Sprinkle with pepper and salt.
4. Take out of the skillet and add the walnuts. Toss to combine.

Garlicky Green Beans

This recipe makes 4 servings and contains 104 calories; 9 grams fat; 4 grams protein; 1 gram net carbohydrates per serving

What You Need

- Grated Parmesan, .25 c

- Olive oil, 2 tbsp.

- Pepper

- Salt

- Minced garlic, 1 tsp.

- Steamed green beans, 1 lb.

What to Do

1. You need to warm your oven to 425.

2. Lay some parchment on a cooking sheet.

3. Sprinkle with pepper and salt.

4. Spread evenly onto baking sheet. Place into the oven for ten minutes. Beans should be tender and slightly browned.

5. Sprinkle on Parmesan cheese and enjoy.

Creamed Spinach

This recipe makes 4 servings and contains 195 calories; 20 grams fat; 3 grams protein; 1 gram net carbohydrates per serving

What You Need

- Pepper
- Salt
- Nutmeg
- Chicken broth, .25 c
- Heavy cream, .75 c
- Spinach, 4 c
- Thinly sliced small onion
- Butter, 1 tbsp.

What to Do

1. Place a skillet on top of the stove and melt the butter on medium heat.
2. Cook the onions until slightly caramelized around five minutes.
3. Put the nutmeg, pepper, salt, chicken broth, heavy cream, and spinach into the skillet. Stir well to combine.
4. Cook until spinach is tender and sauce is thick. This will take about 15 minutes.

Zucchini Crisps

This recipe makes 4 servings and contains 94 calories; 8 grams fat; 4 grams protein; 1 gram net carbohydrates per serving

What You Need

- Pepper

- Grated Parmesan cheese, .5 c

- Sliced zucchini, 4

- Butter, 2 tbsp.

What to Do

1. Slice the zucchini into round slices that are about a fourth-inch circle.

2. Place a large skillet on top of the stove and melt the butter on medium.

3. Cook the zucchini in the pan, cooking until tender and browned.

4. Sprinkle with Parmesan.

5. Cook until cheese is melted and crispy. This will take an additional five minutes.

Mashed Cheesy Cauliflower

This recipe makes 4 servings and contains 183 calories; 15 grams fat; 8 grams protein; 4 grams net carbohydrates per serving

What You Need

- Pepper
- Salt
- Room temp butter, 2 tbsp.
- Heavy cream, .25 c
- Shredded cheddar, .5 c
- Chopped cauliflower, 1 head

What to Do

1. Place the chopped cauliflower into a saucepan and put water into it that covers the cauliflower.

2. Place on top of the stove and let it come to a boil.

3. Let this boil for five minutes and pour into a colander. Let it drain completely.

4. Place into a food processor and break up into smaller pieces. Add in butter, cream, and cheese. Process until whipped and creamy.

5. Add pepper and salt to taste.

Mushroom and Camembert

This recipe makes 4 servings and contains 161 calories; 13 grams fat; 9 grams protein; 3 grams net carbohydrates per serving

What You Need

- Pepper

- Diced Camembert, 4 oz.

- Halved button mushrooms, 1 lb.

- Minced garlic, 2 tsp.

- Butter, 2 tbsp.

What to Do

1. Place a skillet on top of the stove and melt the butter on medium heat.

2. Place the garlic in the skillet and cook until fragrant.

3. Add mushrooms continue to cook until tender around ten minutes.

4. Add in cheese and cook until melted.

5. Add pepper, taste and adjust seasonings if needed.

Zucchini Noodles with Pesto

This recipe makes 4 servings and contains 93 calories; 8 grams fat; 4 grams protein; 2 grams net carbohydrates per serving

What You Need

- Grated Parmesan cheese, .25 c

- Zucchini, 4

- EVOO, .25 c

- Nutritional yeast, 2 tsp.

- Garlic cloves, 3

- Basil leaves, 1 c

- Chopped kale, 1 c

What to Do

1. Place the yeast, garlic, basil, and kale into a food processor. Process until finely chopped.

2. Keeping the food processor on low, drizzle in the olive oil until it forms a thick paste. Add some water if it gets too thick.

3. Either use a peeler to turn the zucchini into "noodles" or use a spiralizer. Place into a bowl.

4. Stir in pesto and parmesan cheese. Give everything a good toss to get everything coated.

Bacon and Blue Cheese Zoodles

This recipe makes 1 serving, and contains 435 calories; 33 grams fat; 21 grams protein; 5 grams net carbohydrates per serving

What You Need

- Pepper

- Cooked and crumbled bacon, .5 c

- Crumbled blue cheese, .33 c

- Blue cheese dressing, 3 tbsp.

- Baby spinach, .5 cup

- Spiralized zucchini, 1 c

What to Do

1. Put all ingredients into a bowl. Toss well to coat. Serve.

2. If you don't have a spiralizer, you can get the same effect by using a peeler.

Conclusion

Thank you for making it through to the end of the 30-Day Ketogenic Meal Plan. Let's hope it was informative and able to provide you with all of the tools you need to achieve your goals, whatever they may be.

A ketogenic diet is a great way to lose weight and get healthy. With planning and tons of recipes at your disposal, you are sure to be successful. The key to seeing results is to make the diet as easy as possible. Creating a meal plan can do just that. Use the information you have learned in this book to do just that.

Diets don't have to be boring. In fact, the more fun and variety you can have with a diet, the easier it will be. The limitless number of meal plan creations you can make with the recipes found in this book is sure to keep you interested. Don't continue to put off changing the way you eat. Make the change today, and you will see the results.

Finally, if you found this book useful in any way, a review is always appreciated!

www.ingramcontent.com/pod-product-compliance
Lightning Source LLC
Chambersburg PA
CBHW080417030426
42335CB00020B/2485